Lecture Notes of the Institute for Computer Sciences, Social Informatics and Telecommunications Engineering 70

Silvia Gabrielli   Dirk Elias
Kanav Kahol (Eds.)

Ambient Media and Systems

Second International ICST Conference
AMBI-SYS 2011
Porto, Portugal, March 24-25, 2011
Revised Selected Papers

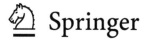 Springer

Volume Editors

Silvia Gabrielli
CREATE-NET
38123 Trento, Italy
E-mail: silvia.gabrielli@create-net.org

Dirk Elias
Fraunhofer Portugal - AICOS
4200-135 Porto, Portugal
E-mail: dirk.elias@fraunhofer.pt

Kanav Kahol
Arizona State University
School of Computing and Informatics
Phoenix, AZ 85004, USA
E-mail: kanav.kahol@asu.edu

ISSN 1867-8211
ISBN 978-3-642-23901-4
DOI 10.1007/978-3-642-23902-1

e-ISSN 1867-822X
e-ISBN 978-3-642-23902-1

Springer Heidelberg Dordrecht London New York

Library of Congress Control Number: 2011935607

CR Subject Classification (1998): H.5, H.4, C.2, I.4, K.4, J.3

Typesetting: Camera-ready by author, data conversion by Scientific Publishing Services, Chennai, India

Printed on acid-free paper

Springer is part of Springer Science+Business Media (www.springer.com)

Preface

Ambi-sys 2011, the Second International Conference on Ambient Systems and Media, was held in Casa da Musica, Porto, during March 24-25, 2011.

The conference focus was on emerging technologies, services and solutions for new, human-centric ambient environments. It aimed at bringing together international senior and junior researchers, as well as developers and industry delegates to discuss issues and trends, research and technological advances in the area of design and deployment of ambient systems and media.

The conference was structured as a single-track, multi-session event. To encourage active participation and the potential formation of new collaborations among attendees, the atmosphere was kept informal. This was also helped by the original and inspirational conference venue of Casa da Musica, which represents today a cultural meeting point in the city of Porto, providing an ideal space for different types of artists and knowledge creators to interact with their audiences.

Contributions to the conference were solicited in the form of full and short research papers and workshop proposals. After a thorough review process of the papers received, for which we thank the Technical Program Committee, ten were accepted for the main conference and one as a workshop proposal.

This was eventually organized as a thematic session on the topic of Advanced Materials and Creative Design Thinking for Ambient Intelligence, moderated by Raymond Oliver (Northumbria University, UK) and Anne Toomey (Royal College of Art, UK), which opened the conference. During this session all delegates were invited to participate in brainstorming and in-depth discussions on the opportunities offered by new materials, such as active polymers, to inspire innovative solutions in the field of ambient assisted living, providing a new physical basis for ambient intelligence by also leveraging on contributions offered by interaction design methods and approaches.

On behalf of the Organizing Committee of Ambi-sys 2011, we would like to thank ICST and Create-Net for technical sponsorship of the event. A special thanks also to the volunteer efforts of the Fraunhofer AICOS group and Susana Hotz, in particular, for their local support and endless patience.

Last but not least, we would like to thank all the authors who submitted papers, making the conference possible, and the authors of accepted papers for their valuable contribution.

Silvia Gabrielli
Dirk Elias
Kanav Kahol

Organization

Steering Committee

Imrich Chlamtac   President of Create-Net, Italy

Conference General Chair

Kanav Kahol   Arizona State University, USA

Technical Program Chair

Silvia Gabrielli   Create-Net, Italy

Local Chair

Dirk Elias   Fraunhofer Portugal Research Center for Assistive Information and Communication Solutions FhP-AICOS, Portugal

Workshop Chair

Winslow Burleson   Arizona State University, USA

Publicity Chair

Constantinos T. Angelis   Technological Educational Institute of Epirus, Greece

Panel Chair

Pedro Santos   Fraunhofer IGD, Germany

Web Chair

Mithra Vankipuram   Arizona State University, USA

Conference Coordinator

Aza Swedin   European Alliance for Innovation (EAI)

Technical Program Committee

Anthony Jameson	DFKI, Germany
Tiziana Catarci	University of Rome La Sapienza, Italy
Raquel Navarro-Prieto	BarcelonaMedia, Spain
Oswald Lanz	FBK-irst, Italy
Huzur Saran	IIT Delhi, India
Kumar Rajamani	Amrita University, India
Oscar Mayora	Create-Net, Italy
William Hazlewood	Indiana University, USA
Margarita Anastassova	CEA, France
Nuno Otero	University of Minho, Portugal
Baoxin Li	Arizona State University, USA
Panagiotis Demestichas	University of Piraeus, Greece
Patrik Floreen	Helsinki Institute for Information Technology HIIT, Finland
Ivan Lee	Ryerson University, Canada
Venet Osmani	Create-Net, Italy
Stefan Arbanowski	Fraunhofer Fokus, Germany
Matthieu Boussard	Alcatel Lucent Bell Labs, USA
Ben Falchuk	Telcordia Technologies Inc., USA
Ramiro Velazquez	Universidad Panamericana, Mexico
Ralf Kernchen	University of Surrey, UK
Vera Stavroulaki	University of Piraeus, Greece
Junaid Chaudhry	University of Hail, Saudi Arabia

Table of Contents

Session 4

Session 5

A Physical Basis for Ambient Intelligence

The Convergence of Biology, Polymers and Electronics Enabling New Design Approaches to Assistive Living

Raymond Oliver[1] and Anne Toomey[2]

[1] Northumbria University School of Design
Squires Building, Sandyford Road Newcastle NE1 8ST, United Kingdom
raymond.oliver@northumbria.ac.uk
[2] Deputy Head, Department of Textiles, Royal College of Art
Kensington Gore, London SW7 2EU, United Kingdom
anne.toomey@rca.ac.uk

Abstract. Innovation in materials drives new technologies - in the 1930's DuPont and ICI discovered and developed Nylon and Polyethylene polymerisation. Today, a new wave of conjugated conductive polymers is emerging, with electronic properties akin to Silicon with effects & interactions stemming from the electronic configuration within the material allowing them to be programmed, through their electron mobility, yielding conformable logic and memory devices. These active polymers are flexible, lightweight, transparent and solution processable, lending themselves to applications and opportunities in ambient assisted living, driving printed electronics and optoelectronics. This paper outlines the principles and provides initial examples of studies underway afforded by the physical basis for ambient intelligence, pursued through a P^3i Design Research Studio.

Keywords: Ambient intelligence, organic electronics, assistive living, creative design, design-science interactions.

1 Introduction

Ambient Intelligence (AmI) has emerged from ubiquitous/pervasive computing and the virtual 'internet of things' to a more tangible physical basis which, in general, follows Weisser's definition of human centred/needs driven technologies incorporating healthcare, convenience, information access, connectivity and generally making life simpler and more stress free [1]. The new drivers accelerating an ambient life environment are the emergence of conformable conjugated conductive polymers, i.e. electro, photo and bio active, capable of designed development to incorporate into objects, devices and interactive consumer products. Organic macro electronics

S. Gabrielli, D. Elias, and K. Kahol (Eds.): AMBI-SYS 2011, LNICST 70, pp. 1–11, 2011.
© Institute for Computer Sciences, Social Informatics and Telecommunications Engineering 2011

began to make AmI into the embedded 'visible invisibility', anticipated in the mid 90's and made into physical reality by the wave of new nanomaterials and active polymers now emerging. Combining information, intuition and intelligent structures, they bring about the missing link in most analyses of AmI that is the creation of a processable and implementable physical basis for ambient assisted life technologies and applications. The physicality of ambient intelligence is a 'killer application' that will also drive sustainable printable consumer electronics and will be a significant factor in the uptake of nanotechnology [3]. What is the best way to use ambient intelligence and in what ways can it enhance the way we live? On starting to scrutinise the current facts it quickly becomes apparent that this is an interesting and exciting challenge. To examine what is intended by ambient intelligence and what will be its potential consequences is important contribution to the development of a calmer society, to more satisfied consumers and accelerating a printed electronics future.

2 Disruptive Technologies and the Emergence of AmI Environments

A common barrier to sustaining a high rate of growth in any industry is the existence of fundamental limitation to the basic technologies on which the industry depends. Improvements are instead evolutionary in nature and focussed largely around operating cost reduction. However, by contrast, no fundamental limitation in the technologies enabling the semi-conductor industry has yet arisen as a significant barrier to its continued growth. Beyond 2016 and the demise of the 'top-down' lithographic technologies employed, 'bottom-up' nanomaterials fabrication for nano-electronics have the potential to move electronic materials, computers and devices into a new era of sustainable growth. There are still so many opportunities for further improvements in electronics technology, the question of whether it will continue to enjoy rapid growth depends on a different consideration – will the potential new applications that can be supported by increasingly capable electronics technology fulfil a societal need? Will there be a new application area, like the PC or mobile phone to restore high growth to the industry? Ambient Intelligence is the most obvious candidate. It has the potential to fulfil a significant societal need – the need to simplify human interactions with the plethora of electronic devices that surround us today and take advantage of the unfulfilled capabilities of electronic devices to make life easier and more productive through ubiquitous access to information and knowledge. If this technology is widely accepted and adapted, it will certainly establish rapid and sustainable growth in the electronics industry. The concept likely to gain a significant degree of acceptance of this technology is its potential to improve the quality of our lives. Figure 1.

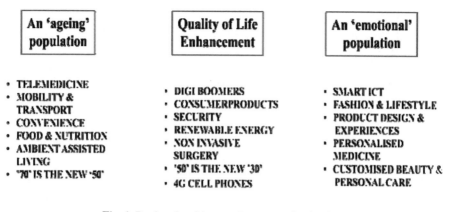

An 'ageing' population	Quality of Life Enhancement	An 'emotional' population
• TELEMEDICINE • MOBILITY & TRANSPORT • CONVENIENCE • FOOD & NUTRITION • AMBIENT ASSISTED LIVING • '70' IS THE NEW '50'	• DIGI BOOMERS • CONSUMERPRODUCTS • SECURITY • RENEWABLE ENERGY • NON INVASIVE SURGERY • '50' IS THE NEW '30' • 4G CELL PHONES	• SMART ICT • FASHION & LIFESTYLE • PRODUCT DESIGN & EXPERIENCES • PERSONALISED MEDICINE • CUSTOMISED BEAUTY & PERSONAL CARE

Fig. 1. Putting the citizen at the centre of technology

3 Ambient Intelligence Origins

As a key element of the physical AmI concept, the computers recede into the background. AmI at its most effective will engage only the periphery of our attention and engage the centre of our attention only when the 'visible invisibility' situation demands it. A 'calm technology' will enhance our peripheral reach by bringing more details into the perception, making us feel at home in a comfortable space. Model systems examples include the automobile, the airplane and the built environment. By contrast, the current generation of PC's and other personal electronic devices are not 'calm' but at the centre of our attention when we interact with them [4].

3.1 Ambient Intelligence Development

AmI, emerging in the 1990's, presents a vision for 'soft' electronic technologies from 2010 onwards. Lighting, sound vision, domestic appliances personal healthcare devices, furniture, interior walls / surfaces and distributed services all cooperate seamlessly with one another to improve the total use experience through the support of natural and intuitive interfaces. Ambient intelligence builds on mobile and pervasive computing and refers to electronic systems that are sensitive and responsive to the presence of people. 'Ambient' here refers to the need for a large scale embedding of technology; 'intelligence' refers to the digital surroundings exhibiting specific forms of social interaction. By implication, embedding through miniaturisation and novel direct write techniques is the systems design objective from a hardware point of view. For software, the main objective is to introduce true intelligence into the systems [1], [4]. One of the most significant conclusions from the field of embedded technology is that the design and manufacture of electronic devices has indeed reached a level of miniaturisation, transparency and conformability allowing integration of electronic systems (organic CMOS) for processing, communicating, storage display and access into any possible physical object, like clothes, furniture, cars and homes – thus making peoples environments 'smart'. This

this recent discovery, described below, will accelerate and enhance the ubiquitous take-up of AmI and is the basis for driving many aspects of plastic electronic applications.

3.2   System + Social + Cognitive Intelligence

The AmI vision has human needs as the key element in the development of digital innovations, while technology is seen as a means to achieve this objective. Aspects such as information overload, violations of privacy and a lack of control and trustworthiness in general, threaten the introduction of novel technologies into our everyday lives and consequently, it is often not clear whether people will perceive such scenarios as beneficial. Essential are the user experiences perceived when interacting with AmI environments. Examples of such experiences are immersion in social connectivity, viewed as emergent features of intelligent behaviour in AmI systems. The system intelligence drivers i.e. context awareness, personalisation, adaptive behaviour and anticipation, primarily facilitate intelligent communication with AmI environments, thus providing users with a means for intelligent interaction and control. With the increased expectations of AmI technologies, the true intelligence of AmI environments requires complying with societal conventions and with cognitive intelligence, allowing for sensory and emotional experiences and judgements [6], [7].

3.3   Materials Intelligence and the Rise of Electro and Photo Active Conductive Polymers

To meet many of the above criteria, materials and devices are needed that are physically unobtrusive, embedded in the common environments of the everyday. The crucial breakthrough in materials came in the 1980's and can now drive AmI forward. These materials are known as OFEDs – organic, flexible electronic devices. OFEDs are derived from a molecular engineering approach to create an intelligent materials platform. Solution processed OFEDs are attractive and it is now possible to envision a high throughput reel to reel (R2R) printing process to make large area OFEDs at low cost. Possible techniques for high throughput large area printing are screen, gravure or flexography The heart of the design paradigm for solution processable OFEDs technology lies in adding as much functionality as possible into the active organic materials and then use these materials in device structures with as few active layers as possible. Scaling solution processable technology for large area OFEDs requires the development of new solution based processes. To do this systematically requires a deep knowledge of the behaviour and characteristics of both polymeric and small molecule organic semiconductors. Over the last three years, such materials driven technology has reached demonstrable scales of operation compatible with realistic testing for ambient intelligent applications [8]. The reason for these developments is the fact that many of the new functional materials are solution processable. As mentioned previously, the classes of material which are becoming available are derivatives of the original discoveries made by Heeger et al [10] in the late 70's based on conjugated, conductive polymers and by Friend et al [11] in the early 1980's based on light emitting polymers - in other words, conformable, lightweight, transparent electro and photo active polymeric and to a lesser extent, small molecule organic materials. When we couple these to:

a)   creative design principles and techniques and
b)   assistive human benefits through medicine, transport, shelter, information, communication

then we create both a needs driven and market driven set of drivers, accelerating the implementation of processes to make AmI environments at the most economical cost, while providing valuable functionality and/or experiences [9]. A major benefit, which impacts the uptake of OFEDs, is the fact that many of the 'active' materials can be synthesised in the form of polymeric and gel solutions. This flexibility, in a phase transformation such as a chemical reaction, a cross linkage step, a solidification, a drying or a curing step, allow the transition of bulk fluid to controllable physical forms [12] i.e.

a)   Droplet and spray production ('dots')
b)   Fibre spinning & material phase transformation ('lines')
c)   Thin film, multilayer extrusion & deposition ('surfaces')
d)   Rapid Prototyping - 3^D printing & injection moulding ('structures')

These methodologies allow designers much greater flexibility to create the desired 2D & 3 D materials and to experiment with multiple composite forms previously untried, if given ample quantities of material [13].

e)   'Dots': planar, sheet to sheet printing, using DoD ink jet for small & large area applications (cm^2)
f)   'Lines': fibres (weaving, knitting, sewing & embroidery) for relatively large area applications ($m^{2)}$
g)   'Surfaces': large area screen printing, Reel To Reel web based printing and multilayer, thin film extrusion for very large area applications (km^2)!

On Body Applications
a)   Clothes & Fashion: light, sound, sensory effects in location/mood context
b)   Healthcare: point of care diagnostics based on bio sensors in clothing. Patient care – chronic wound monitoring, therapeutic response and data reading & analysis
c)   Personal/Beauty care: controlled release materials with smart environmental triggers for sensory, body temperature and antibacterial benefit.

Around Body Applications
a)   Transportation: Organic pixelated lighting, controlled by the driver's and passenger's state of tiredness, need for information etc. Bio sensing of both people and environment integrated into sensory responsive hydrogels

b) Built environment: Smart furniture, interior walls, carpets and curtains, draperies, provide information on an individual basis, using RFID / Bluetooth signalling and large area ultralow cost sensor driveways. Smart health sensing, for both the inhabitants and the fabric, of the living space
c) Renewable energy: Large area portable (power) storage and hence low cost heating and lighting into off grid living environments

4 New Research Perspectives

AmI development and implementation is relatively still in its infancy. As with most disruptive concepts, this is primarily due to the gap that exists between the fiction of the conceptual vision on the one hand and the intricacy of the realisation on the other. The factors which influence the speed of uptake can be distinguished as follows [14], [15]:

4.1   Ambient Control (AmC)

To access and control devices in an AmI environment, the issue is integrating the physical world into the digital world with functionalities like sensing, actuation, identification and secure (wireless) access, collecting and interpreting information about objects and their surroundings. It should support context, meaning, sensory effects and semantics. AmI should also support the distribution of media over physical devices, to integrate virtual and physical worlds and enable the distribution of media onto physical objects, supporting combinations of the senses: audio, video, lighting, fragrance and vibration through to distributed media services. This is what Aarts calls the extension of 'Quality of Service' (QoS) into the concept of 'Quality of Experience' (QoE) [6]. To provide ambient control, a standardised open platform is needed. A promising approach could well be the 'internet of things', a novel use of the current internet, aiming at serving and activation through URLs and quality controlled access layers i.e. access to physical layers, surfaces and interfaces. The interactive nature of these surfaces and interfaces can now be realised with active fabrics and non-woven thin films that can be designed and incorporated into many everyday objects.

4.2   Sensory Experiences

To process information in the interaction with AmI environments, the issue is to understand the interaction between the human brain and its environment. This field is concerned with the investigation of fundamental and essential functions of the brain, including perception, thinking, emotion, learning, memory, attention, heuristic search, reasoning, discovery, creativity and surprise [7], Figure 2.
    Key elements are the measurement of the emotional and mental state of the users in a reliable way and using this information to enhance the interaction with AmI environments. Capturing, influencing and generating emotions is a new field of research and is often referred to as 'affective' computing. Key questions include:

how can we model a mood state? Which moods do we need to be able to capture? How does triggering a set of senses influence the perceived emotions? Sensing and actuation of sensorial effects in relation to human activity are important elements in the development of effective solutions in sensory experiences [16].

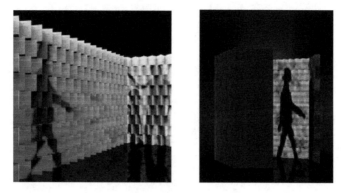

Fig. 2. Looking through a concrete wall, light transmitting concrete blocks embedded with luminous glass fibres. ©Litracon

4.3   New e-Inclusion

What does it take for people to accept that their environment is monitoring their every move, waiting for the right moment to take over the purpose of taking care of them? Much of the acceptance will depend on the perceived functional benefit of AmI environments and on the availability of mechanisms that enable participants to make their own choices in a way that is understandable, transparent and independent of their comprehension level.

4.4   Ethical Concerns

Personalisation requires registration and recording of the user behaviour. The explicit knowledge about the so-called 'digital soul' of human beings requires the development of different standards for social behaviour and it might even be desired to protect people against their own attitudes. Ethical concern is given to the possibility to incorporate AmI into the human body. We are already incorporating intelligence into our clothing and we are happy to have a pacemaker built in. Targeted drug delivery or minimally invasive surgery approaches are medical treatments based on embedded electronics; evidently, this has a medical justification.

5   Northumbria University School of Design / Royal College of Art Activities

Over the last two years we have been examining the interactive factors that are required to create and interpret aspects of human centred needs that constitute ambient assistive technology of sustainable value. In addition to those factors which have been well documented in the literature, i.e. system and social intelligence [2], we can only move towards a robust physical basis for AmI if we have at our disposal new, innovative materials with appropriate molecular and electronic structures. Conjugated, conductive polymers integrated with nanoscalar materials yield a sound

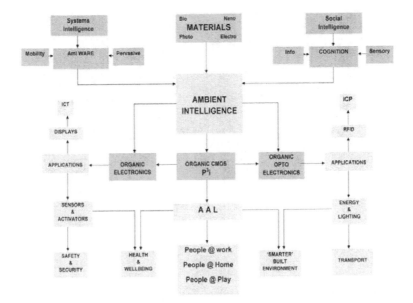

Fig. 3. Northumbria / RCA template to advance the Design – AmI interface

platform for the physicality of AmI and hence beneficial applications in ambient assisted living. Figure 3 above details the mapping process we are using to plot a path towards physical AmI based on electro, photo and even bio active and responsive polymers and gels. A crucial element is the solution processability of these materials that allows deposition and/or embedding into almost any surface shape [17]. The future goal of the work is to develop 'Active' Materials for Life design research hub, to explore the deployment of physical AmI through needs driven applications in assistive health, transport, the built environment and interactive consumer products [18].

5.1   Design: STEM Explorations in Physical Ambient Intelligence Environments

Much has been written on the development of HCI and 'smart' environments. All are based on the use of Silicon semiconductor technology to provide programmable environments. The recent growth and interest in organic conductive polymers mentioned earlier allows further advances to be made on three fronts:

a) Solution processable, transparent conductive polymers which are printable, paintable and programmable, i.e. organic CMOS
b) Such materials are transparent, lightweight and conformable and are thus capable of creative design development
c) Beyond the ability to code electro and photoactive conjugated conductive polymers and stimuli responsive gels, biopolymers and shape memory alloys yield substantially greater bandwidth in terms of physical and emotional actions.

5.2   An 'Active' Materials for Living Platform [AMfL]

As examples, we are investigating aspects of a), b) and c) in a joint interactive design research studio P^3i (paintable, printable, programmable materials) environment with contributions from textiles and fashion design, industrial design, materials chemistry, systems biology, chemical nanotechnology and printed electronics based hardware design.   This skill set forms the basis for the P^3i interdisciplinary design research centre at NUSDL and is focussed on an 'Active Materials for Living' platform with the work programme pillars: SENE, BIOSYS, AMBIENT and KNIT.

SENSE: Smart, Sustainable Multisensory Material Design. This pillar focuses on mental wellness and sleep disorder by delivering effective new ways to improve emotional wellbeing.Fusing design-led wearable technologies that sense the human condition with aromachology research, new product focus can be generated which dispense as 'casket' of fragrances to influence moods or emotional states in different situations.   The programme of design research includes the development of wearable technology and responsive jewellery as convenient delivery vehicles for fragrance 'bubbles'.

BIOSYS. Biosys is an explanation of the benefits which can be achieved through the convergence of biology-polymers-electronics and the use of printed systems technology to create a bridge between sensing, bio mimicry and responsive materials, in particular, the creation of bio-textiles as wearable technology with suitable properties activated by chemical sensing and actuation. Another focus is on sustainable bio fibre and fabric production through novel biological processes; applications for bio responsive and bio compatible fabrics lie in transportation and architecture as well as in sustainable textiles for fashion.

The above two pillars relate to systems biology, printable sensing and novel product fabrication technologies towards organic ambient environments.

AMBIENT & KNIT. Both of these projects focus on the emergence of organic CMOS to provide a physical basis for Ambient Intelligence (AmI) through conformable and often transparent active materials integrated with printable sensing. The focus is on science & design in society, embedding intelligence into social environments in three areas of life quality:

a)   Assets in Life (home, the car, furniture, interiors, clothes)
b)   Phases in Life (childhood, youth, parenthood, old age)
c)   Aspects of Life (learning, sleeping, eating, connecting, networking)

The materials and technologies to create 'visible invisibility' are being examined through specific ways of creating AmI in either everyday objects or through some of the wearable technologies.

6   Conclusions and Final Remarks

Substantial technological and societal barriers to the full implementation of AmI are described by Weisser [1] and by Aarts   [6]. They even push implementation into the distant future, but partial implementation, designed to make life easier and improve the effectiveness of work processes without threatening privacy and freedom of action, is likely. Another partial implementation route is centred on RFID where the possible applications include full implementation of AmI. Applications relating to retail, security, transportation, manufacturing and shipping are users of RFID tags produced in high volumes at very low cost and are a significant user of plastic electronics capability today. In the full integration of physical AmI, wearable electronics or 'smart' textiles on clothing are an important element in ambient intelligence computing, communication and I/O interface implementation. Conversely, in the absence of success with AmI it is doubtful that wearable electronics will result in anything beyond novelty items. However, novelty should never be underestimated as an early driver for the uptake of new products. In addition to novelty, the needs of the military and security sectors and of haute couture are significant drivers for wearable electronics, wearable light and also wearable (and disposable) power and is well illustrated by the work of Suzanne Kuechler (at UCL) works on materials culture & communication to enhance aesthetics & functionality [19]. If implementation is done well, all of these elements will work together as a calm technology, reducing the current clutter of activities that we expect as part of the work environment [20]. It is not likely that ambient intelligence implementations would be just as visualized by Weisser. This emanates from the proven inability of anyone, however brilliant, to predict the future of technology. It will not be a surprise if ambient intelligence is highly successful, but the eventual implementation will certainly be different in important ways from that presently visualised. The basis for physical AmI is now available through the use of electro, photo and bioactive polymers and gels, which are solution processable. To ensure a reasonable and sustainable uptake of AmI to improve the quality of peoples' lives, a number of key materials and tools need to be in place:

a)   Innovative display fabrication
b)   Useful opto electronics
c)   Miniaturised micro and nano printed sensors and actuators
d)   Integrating much of the above into a creative design platform

References

1. Weisser, M.: The computer for the 21st century. Scientific American, 94–100 (1991)
2. Aarts, E.H.L., Ouwarkerk, M. (eds.): AmIware: Hardware drivers for Ambient Intelligence. Springer, Berlin (2005)

3. Royal Society, Royal Academy of Engineering, Nanoscience and nanotechnologies. Royal Society, London (2004)
4. Denning, J. (ed.): The Invisible Future. McGraw Hill, New York (2001)
5. Aarts, E.H.L., Encarnacao, J.: True visions: The emergence of Ambient Intelligence. Springer, Berlin (2006)
6. Aarts, E.H.L., Diederiks, E.: Ambient Lifestyle: From concepts to experience. BIS, Amsterdam (2007)
7. Petkovic, M., Jonker, W. (eds.): Privacy & trust in modern data management. Springer, Berlin (2007)
8. Klauk, H. (ed.): Organic electronics: Materials, manufacturing and applications. Wiley VCH, Weinheim (2006)
9. Addington, M., Schodek, D.: Smart materials and technologies. Elsevier Architectural Press, Oxford (2004)
10. Heeger, A., et al.: Physical Review Letters 39, 1098 (1977) et seq
11. Friend, R., et al.: Nature 347, 539 (1990) et seq
12. Oliver, R., Tillotson, J., Toomey, A.: Nanoengineered textiles and nonwovens using electro and photo active polymers. J. of Fibre, Bioengineering and Informatics 2(1) (2009)
13. Oliver, R., Toomey, A.: Innovating for the future. In: Proceedings of Smart Fabrics Conference, Rome (2009)
14. Cai, Y., Abascal, J. (eds.): Ambient Intelligence in everyday lives. Springer, Berlin (2006)
15. Aarts, E.H.L., Marzano, S. (eds.): The New Everyday: Visions of Ambient Intelligence. OIO Publishing, Rotterdam (2003)
16. Tillotson, J., Jenkins, G.: Scent whisper. In: Proceedings IET Seminar on MEMS
17. Oliver, R., Toomey, A.: Design drives materials innovation. Ingenia, Journal of Royal Academy of Engineering (42) (2009)
18. Davies, M., Rogers, R.: A wall for all seasons. RIBA Journal, 55–58 (February 1981)
19. Kuechler, S.: Technological materiality: Beyond the dualist paradigm' Theory. Culture & Society 25(1), 101–120 (2008)
20. Gajovic, E.E., Forster, F.: A review of emerging sensor and actuator printable technologies. Biosensors and Bioelectronics 19, 417–422 (2003)

Service Composition and Advanced User Interfaces in the Home of Tomorrow: The SM4All Approach

Tiziana Catarci, Claudio Di Ciccio, Vincenzo Forte, Ettore Iacomussi,
Massimo Mecella, Giuseppe Santucci, and Giuseppe Tino

SAPIENZA – Università di Roma,
Dipartimento di Informatica e Sistemistica ANTONIO RUBERTI
Via Ariosto 25, Roma, Italy
{catarci,cdc,mecella,santucci}@dis.uniroma1.it,
name.surname@gmail.com

Abstract. Houses of tomorrow will be equipped with many sensors, actuators and devices, which collectively will expose services. Such services, composed in an automatic way, and invokable through adaptive user interfaces, can support human inhabitants in their daily activities. In this paper we present the approach and some results of the SM4ALL EU project (http://www.sm4all-project.eu/), which is investigating automatic services composition and advanced user interfaces applied to domotics.

Keywords: SM4ALL, smart devices, advanced user interfaces, service composition, domotics.

1 Introduction

Embedded systems, i.e., specialized computers used in larger systems to control equipment are nowadays pervasive in immersive realities, i.e., scenarios in which, invisibly, they need to continuously interact with human users, in order to provide continuous sensed information and to react to service requests from the users themselves. Examples are digital libraries and eTourism, automotive, next generation buildings and domotics. Sensors/devices/appliances/actuators offering services are no more static, as in classical networks, (e.g., for environmental monitoring and management or surveillance), but they form an overall distributed system that needs to continuously adapt. That can be done by adding, removing and composing on-the-fly basic elements that are the offered services.

This paper intends to outline some insights stemming from the European-funded project SM4ALL (Smart hoMes for All - http://www.sm4all-project. eu/), started on September 1st, 2008 and finishing on August 31st, 2011. SM4ALL aims at studying and developing an innovative platform for software smart embedded services in immersive environments, based on a service-oriented approach and composition techniques. This is applied to the challenging scenario

S. Gabrielli, D. Elias, and K. Kahol (Eds.): AMBI-SYS 2011, LNICST 70, pp. 12–19, 2011.

of private home and building in presence of users with different abilities and needs (e.g., young, elderly or disabled people).

In order to introduce the novel idea of services underlying SM4ALL, the reader should consider the following scenario: a person is at home and decides to take a bath. He/she would like to simply express this to the house and have the available services collaborate in order to move the house itself to a new state which represents the desired one. The temperature in the bathroom is raised through the heating service, the wardrobe in the sleeping room is opened in order to offer the bathrobe, the bath is filled in with 37 °C water, etc. If we suppose the person is a disabled one, some services cannot be directly automated, e.g., the one of helping the person to move into the bath. In this case, a service still exists, but it is offered by a human, e.g., the nurse, which is doing her job in another room, and that at the right moment is notified – through her PDA or any other device – to go into the bath and help the patient. Maybe this service is offered also by the son of the patient (or any other person), living in a nearby house, which is notified at the right moment, and if the nurse is not present at home, to help the patient. The scenario shows the idea of a system of services, some offered in a completely automated way through sensors/appliances/actuators, other realized through the collaboration of other persons, which moves continuously from a desired state to a new one, in order to satisfy user goals. Clearly, as in all complex systems, there are trade-offs to be considered (the goal of the person willing a relaxing bath is in contrast with the availability of the nurse/son offering the "help" service).

The rest of the paper is organized as follows: Section 2 does very briefly provide a background on the current state of the art for home automation systems, Section 3 gives the reader an overview of the SM4ALL system architecture. For sake of space, the remainder of the paper then focuses only on two components, namely the User Interface (Section 4) and the Composition Layer (Section 5), which are among the most innovative ones produced by the project. Finally, the Section 6 draws some conclusions.

2 Relevant Work

Presently, we are assisting at a blooming of research projects on the use of smart services at home and domotics, in particular for assisting people with physical or mental disabilities.

For instance, at Georgia Tech a domotic home has been built for the elder adult with the goals of compensating physical decline, memory loss and supporting communication with relatives [9]. This work also considers issues of acceptability of domotics identifying key issues for the adoption of the technology by the end user. Acceptability, dangers and opportunities are also surveyed in [13]. Having a reliable system is a primary concern for all users.

At Carnegie Mellon people's behavior is studied by automatic analysis of video images [4]. This is fundamental in detecting anomalies and pathologies in a nursing home where many patients live. Pervading the environment with active landmarks, called Cyber Crumbs, aims at guiding the blind by equipping him/her with a smart badge [14]. A number of projects to give virtual companion's to people, to monitor people's health and behavioral patterns, to help Alzheimer patients are presented in [6]. The Gator Tech Smart House [5] is a programmable approach to smart homes targeting the elder citizen. The idea is to have a service layer based on OSGi [15] in order to enable service discovery and composition.

Finally, in [10], the current adoption of service technologies for smart energy systems, including domotic ones, is discussed.

3 The SM4All Architecture

Devices and sensors available in the house constitute the basis of the SM4ALL system. There is an ever increasing variety of devices, for example for controlling parts of the home (doors, lights), or media devices, etc. Sensors are devices for measuring physical quantities, ranging from simple thermometers to self-calibrating satellite-carried radiometers. Sensors and devices have an inherent connection, e.g., a device for opening the window blinds can change the luminosity value sensed by a sensor. Both sensors and devices make their functionalities available according to the service oriented paradigm. In particular, services (offered by sensors and devices) are offered as SOAP-based services, both in the UPnP technology and in the WSDL-based one.

A *Pervasive Controller* is in charge, when a new sensor/device joins the system, to dynamically load and deploy the appropriate service wrapping it, and to register all the relevant information into the *Service Repository*. Each service, in order to be dynamically configurable and composable, exposes rich service descriptions, comprising *(i)* interface specifications, *(ii)* specifications of the externally visible behaviors, *(iii)* offered QoS. As previously introduced, human actors in the environment are also abstracted as services, and actually "wrapped" with a rich description (e.g., a nurse offering medical services). This allows including them in a service composition and having them collaborate with devices and sensors to reach a certain goal. Such rich service descriptions are stored in the Service Repository, in order to be queried and retrieved by the other components of the architecture. During their operation, services continuously change their status, both in terms of values of sensed/actuating variables (e.g., a service wrapping a temperature sensor report the current sensed temperature, a service wrapping windows blinds report whether the blinds are open, closed, half-way, etc.) and in terms of conversational state of the service itself. All these status information are available, through a publish&subscribe mechanism, in the *Context Manager*.

On the basis of the rich service descriptions, a *Composition Engine* is in charge of providing complex services by suitably composing available ones. The engine can work in two different ways: *(i)* off-line and *(ii)* on-line. In the off-line mode, at design/deployment time of the house, a desiderata (i.e., not really existing) target service is defined, and the composition engine (through its synthesis subcomponent) synthesizes a suitable orchestration of the available services realizing the target one. Such an orchestration specification is used at execution-time (i.e., when the user chooses to invoke the composite/desiderata service) by the orchestration subcomponent in order to coordinate the available services (i.e., to interact with the user on one hand and to schedule service invocations on the other hand). In this mode, the orchestration specification is synthesized off-line (i.e., not during user requests) and executed on-line as if it were a real service of the home. The off-line mode is technically based on the so-called Roman approach to automatic service composition [1]. Conversely in the on-line mode, the user, during its interaction with the home, may decide not to invoke a specific service (either available/real or composite one), but to ask the home to realize a goal; in such a case, the composition engine, on the basis of specific planning techniques [8], synthesizes and executes available service invocations in order to reach such a goal.

The user is able to interact with the home through different kinds of *user interfaces*, either centralized (e.g., in a home control station accessible through a touchscreen in the living room) or distributed and embedded in specific interface devices. Specifically, Brain Computer Interfaces (BCIs) allow also people with disabilities to interact with the system.

4   The User Interface

The home can be controlled from the user through different kinds of interfaces (BCIs, remote controls, touch screens, keyboards, voice recognition, etc.). The *AAI* (Abstract Adaptive Interface) represents the core of the SM4ALL user layer. It retrieves status information from the Context Manager and the service descriptions from the Service Repository and organizes everything in order to correctly show available actions to the user, depending on the interaction mode she is currently making use of (i.e., visual, aural, BCI, etc.). The AAI is intended indeed to be put as an abstraction layer among the multiple user interface devices and the underlying composition layer.

Its main novelty is represented by the ability to manage many different user interface models with a unique adaptable algorithm, able to change itself on the basis of the interaction device characteristics (speech/aural, visual/touch, handheld, brain-controlled...) and on the basis of the user preferences, automatically gathered, analyzed and synthesized on top of the previous interactions with the system.

Through a message screen the user can see notifications coming from the system. The room actions' screen shows the list of actions that can be invoked, gathered up by groups which are built according to the rooms where the services offering the actions are actually located. The number of available services in the home can be very high, and a service can offer many actions; on the other hand, the icons that can be shown on a screen is limited. A pagination of the information, though useful and indeed exploited in many prototypes, is not sufficient to provide an effective interaction, since it would introduce a huge effort for the user to find the desired element among the big amount of items, navigating back and forth. Hence, in SM4ALL, the AAI integrates a mechanism for grouping and smartly ordering the icons in order to improve the ease of interaction. An icon may represent either a service or an action. Sometimes, only a few actions, among the ones offered by a given service, are available, e.g., a "bedroom light" service offers a "turn off" and a "turn on" action, but only the first (or the second, conversely) is available when the lamp is switched on (off). In such a case, there is no need to show the service icon, as the available action is enough.

When the user can fire more than one action, related to a single service, a clustering is needed. It is realized by initially showing the service icon; once activated, all of the other items are hidden and only the available related actions are displayed.

Another way to reduce the number of displayed icons is to divide services themselves into groups represented by a given type (e.g., "Multimedia" for TVs, MP3 players, etc.). The idea is almost the same: at first, the menu shows only a type which many services belong to, and then, after the type is selected, all of the other items are hidden and the only related services are displayed (see Figure 1).

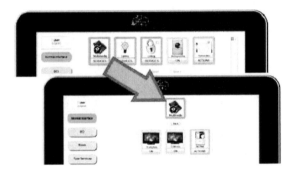

Fig. 1. An example of the user interface grouping services by the type they belong to

Beyond grouping, the AAI exploits the possibility to order the items according to their importance, with respect to the preferences of each user. This way, the actions which are known to be more relevant for the user will be displayed on the first screen, in order to appear at a first glimpse, while the others are going to be shown next. Two algorithms are offered: a *static* one and a *dynamic* one. The user can select which one she prefers through an administration menu. The static algorithm makes use of explicitly defined user settings to identify her preferences. Each preference is constituted by *(i)* a set of conditions, representing the state of the environment which enables the action, *(ii)* a time frame in which the preference has to be considered (Always, Morning, Afternoon, Evening, Night), and *(iii)* a usage expectation degree (certain, highly probable, very probable, probable). The dynamic algorithm orders the actions according to the probability that each one is going to be executed, on the basis of the current environment status and previous invocations: the higher the probability, the higher the priority of the associated icon in the list (*partial order*). The home environment status consists of several parametric values related to the execution (e.g., the 24-hour format time of invocation). Each parameter is associated to a *relevance* (*weight*), manually tunable by administrators. At every call, the parametric value is computed and its *incidence* (*score*) re-calculated. Indeed, it is taken from a run-time updated graph, i.e., a normalized sum of Gaussian curves: at each execution, a new Gaussian centered in the parameter value which is associated to the call (e.g., the time of invocation) is added to the previous graph. In order to tune the evolution of the curve, norm and variance of the Gaussians are both customizable. If the global peak overcomes the maximum admissible value (100%) a normalization is automatically performed (see Figure 2). The probability is thus the *sum* of the *weighted scores* ($\sum_i relevance_i \times incidence_i$) of all the parameters, related to the current home environment status.

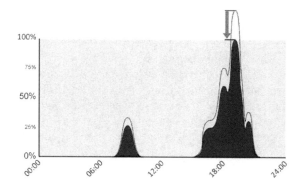

Fig. 2. An example of automatic normalization of the parametric score

5 Composition

The Composition Engine is the component in charge of creating orchestrations which control the whole set of available services spread around the house, in order to satisfy the users' desiderata. It is divided into two different functional components, On-line Synthesis Engine and Off-line Synthesis Engine. As the name suggests, the former performs such a computation at run-time, i.e., as the user asks for a new plan it must return an orchestration to be invoked immediately after. This orchestration is a program that the *Orchestration Engine* must follow step by step in order to achieve the goal. The representation of services is based upon the listing of their pre- and post-conditions, i.e., logic formulae on top of environmental variables such as a room temperature, or light level, which, respectively, *(i)* must be verified for an action to take place and *(ii)* must hold after the action is completed. Goals are logic formulae on top of the same environmental variables, which the user expects to become true due to the enactment of the synthesized plan. The On-line Synthesis Engine reasoning core is a planner that, as described in [7], solves the underlying planning problem through the reduction of it into a CSP (Constraint Satisfaction Problem – see [3]).

In the Off-line Synthesis Engine, services and goals are both descibed by Finite State Automata (FSAs), as in [1]. Goals are target FSAs which the Composition

Engine must realize by simulation, on top of the community of available services. Pre- and post-conditions are expressed as constraints over the FSA transitions (see [11] and [2]), on top of environmental variables. Once the orchestration is computed, the target itself is stored among the community: it can be invoked at any time in the future, like any other service. Such synthesis is fulfilled within a background process by the Composition Engine. The returned orchestration is slightly different from the On-line Synthesis Engine output. Indeed, it is a relation that, given the current target state and the next action to be fired, indicates which services in the community can be invoked in order to enact it, according to any of the possible (i.e., coherent with the realizability of the goal) community and environmental variables states. The Off-line Synthesis Engine solution approach is based on reducing the problem to the synthesis of Linear-time Temporal Logic (LTL) formulae (see [12]) by Model Checking over Game Structures.

The Off-line Synthesis Engine service automaton description language, as well as the orchestration structure definition language, which are used to interact with the component, are XML-based, as a common attitude in service-oriented distributed systems. Their schemata are published under public addresses, so to become a clear interface language not only for the consortium developers but also for external vendors who might want to sell products which are compliant to a SM4ALL standard[1]

As far as the environmental variables are concerned, their types are standardized as well, under a unique data schema. Following the rationale used for services and orchestrations descriptions, it is specified by the definition of hierarchical types in an XML Schema format. Essentially, the SM4ALL data schema imposes a restriction over native XML Schema simple types to limit them to totally ordered countably finite data sets on top of which the developer can define enumerations or intervals, so to make the reasoning over such data feasible[2].

The Repository (see Section 3) is in charge of storing all of XML descriptors. The conversion from such XML formats to internal reasoners input/output formats are up to façade modules which are not exposed to the outside components in the SM4ALL architecture.

6   Concluding Remarks

Throughout this paper, we presented the pervasive intelligent home system SM4ALL, and we focused on the synthesis techniques adopted by its Composition Engine and on the self-adapting ones of the User Interface: they are the components involved the most in the challenge of hiding the heterogeneity of used hardware devices to the other software modules, which is a very important requirement in the field of domotics, where a lack of standardization holds still.

---

[1] The reader can access service and orchestration XML Schemata and related documentation at http://www.dis.uniroma1.it/~cdc/sm4all/proposals/servicemodel/

[2] The reader can find the Schemata and documentation at http://www.dis.uniroma1.it/~cdc/sm4all/proposals/datamodel/

Indeed, this paper also introduces the proposed XML format for the definition of services offered by home devices.

Currently, we are developing a running prototype interfaced with real Konnex, UPnP and Bluetooth devices actually installed in a house set up on purpose in Rome, hosted by Fondazione Santa Lucia. A showcase will be demonstrated in May and October 2011; this will make it possible for us to gather and analyze experimental results in the usage of the new system running.

References

1. Calvanese, D., De Giacomo, G., Lenzerini, M., Mecella, M., Patrizi, F.: Automatic Service Composition and Synthesis: the Roman Model. IEEE Data Eng. Bull. 31(3), 18–22 (2008)
2. De Masellis, R., Di Ciccio, C., Mecella, M., Patrizi, F.: Smart Home Planning Programs. In: Proc. of 2010 International Conference on Service Systems and Service Management (ICSSSM 2010). Japan Advanced Institute of Science and Technology, Japan (2010)
3. Do, M., Kambhampati, S.: Solving Planning-Graph by Compiling it into CSP. In: Proc. AIPS 2000, pp. 82–91 (2000)
4. Hauptmann, A., Gao, J., Yan, R., Qi, Y., Yang, J., Wactlar, H.: Automatic analysis of nursing home observations. IEEE Pervasive Computing 3(2), 15–21 (2004)
5. Helal, S., Mann, W.C., El-Zabadani, H., King, J., Kaddoura, Y., Jansen, E.: The gator tech smart house: A programmable pervasive space. IEEE Computer 38(3), 50–60 (2005)
6. Joseph, A.: Successful aging. IEEE Pervasive Computing 3(2), 36–41 (2004)
7. Kaldeli, E.: Using CSP for Adaptable Web Service Composition. Tech. Rep. 2009-7-01, University of Groningen (2009), www.cs.rug.nl/~eirini/tech_rep_09-7-01.pdf
8. Kaldeli, E., Lazovik, A., Aiello, M.: Extended Goals for Composing Services. In: Proc. 19th International Conference on Automated Planning and Scheduling, ICAPS 2009 (2009)
9. Mynatt, E., Melenhorst, A., Fisk, A., Rogers, W.: Understanding user needs and attitudes. IEEE Pervasive Computing 3(2), 36–41 (2004)
10. Paradiso, J., Dutta, P., Gellersen, H., Schooler, E.: Smart energy systems. special issue. IEEE Pervasive Computing 10 (2011)
11. Patrizi, F.: Simulation-based Techniques for Automated Service Composition. Ph.D. thesis, Department of Systems and Computer Science, SAPIENZA - Universitá di Roma, Rome, Italy (2009)
12. Pnueli, A., Rosner, R.: On the Synthesis of a Reactive Module. In: Proc. POPL, pp. 179–190 (1989)
13. Roberts, J.: Pervasive health management and health management utilizing pervasive technologies: Synergy and issues. The Journal of Universal Computer Science 12(1), 6–14 (2006)
14. Ross, D.: Cyber crumbs for successful aging with vision loss. IEEE Pervasive Computing 3(2), 30–35 (2004)
15. Tuecke, S., Foster, I., Frey, J., Graham, S., Kesselman, C., Maquire, T., Sandholm, T., Snelling, D., Vanderbilt, P.: Open service grid infrastructure (2003)

Wireless Sensor Network Deployment for Building Environmental Monitoring and Control

Essa Jafer[1], Rostislav Spinar[2], Paul Stack[3], Cian O'Mathuna[1], and Dirk Pesch[2]

[1] Tyndall national Institute, Lee Maltings, Prospect Row, Cork, Ireland
[2] Cork Institute of technology (CIT), Cork, Ireland
[3] Department of Civil and Environmental Engineering, University College Cork (UCC), Cork, Ireland
essajh@campus.ie

Abstract. It is commonly agreed that a 15-40% reduction of building energy consumption is achievable by efficiently operated buildings when compared with typical practice. Existing research has identified that the level of information available to Building Managers with existing Building Management Systems and Environmental Monitoring Systems (BMS/EMS) is insufficient to perform the required performance based building assessment. The majority of today's buildings are insufficiently sensored to obtain an unambiguous understanding of performance. The cost of installing additional sensors and meters is extremely high, primarily due to the estimated cost of wiring and the needed labor. From this perspectives wireless sensors technology proves to have a greater cost-efficiency while maintaining high levels of functionality and reliability. In this paper, a wireless sensor network mote hardware design and implementation are introduced for building deployment application. The core of the mote design is based on the 8 bit AVR microcontroller, Atmega1281 and 2.4 GHz wireless communication chip, CC2420. The sensors were selected carefully to meet both the building monitoring and design requirements. Beside the sensing capability, actuation and interfacing to external meters/sensors are provided to perform different management control and data recording tasks. The experiments show that the developed mote works effectively in giving stable data acquisition and owns good communication and power performance.

Keywords: Building automation systems, Wireless Sensor Network, Sensors interfacing and Motes deployment.

1 Introduction

A deeper understanding of system operation is possible if more detailed information is made available to Building Managers. This information must recognize the education and background of Building Managers if they are to fulfill their role with respect to organizational objectives and legislative compliance. Efficiency cannot be determined from displayed sensor readings without data access, storage and post processing. Scheduling information must be displayed concurrently with BMS data. All information used is dependent on accurate, robust and structured data.

S. Gabrielli, D. Elias, and K. Kahol (Eds.): AMBI-SYS 2011, LNICST 70, pp. 20–27, 2011.
© Institute for Computer Sciences, Social Informatics and Telecommunications Engineering 2011

Traditionally building automation systems are realized through wired communications. However, the wired automation systems require expensive communication cables to be installed and regularly maintained and thus they are not widely implemented in industrial plants because of their high cost [1, 2].

In recent years, wireless technologies have become very popular in both home and commercial networking applications. The use of wireless technologies offers distinctive advantages in the field of home and building automation as well [3-5]. First, installation costs are significantly reduced since no cabling is necessary. Neither conduits nor cable trays are required. Wireless technology also allows placing sensors where cabling is not appropriate for aesthetic, conservatory or safety reasons [4, 5]. With current wireless technology, a great challenge arises because of the level of expertise needed to fully make use of the sensors. The most sophisticated hardware often requires advanced knowledge of embedded programming to achieve the level of performance desired. A second issue is about the need for high active lifetime of the wireless installation which means the need for low power design starts with the obligatory use of energy efficient hardware (e.g., low supply voltages and support for sleep modes in microcontrollers) [6].

This paper is focusing on the development of a miniaturized Wireless Sensor platform that intended to be used for building sensing, meters interfacing and actuation. Next the deployment of large scale (around 60 nodes) of this platform was described in terms of network structure, topology and data presentation. The Environmental Research Institute (ERI) building, located at University College Cork (UCC), Ireland was designed as a green flagship building and a low energy research facility [7]. This building was chosen as the test bench for our large scale deployment because it is the most densely measured building on the UCC campus.

2 WSN Node Design

The mote is designed in modular mode. As Fig.1.a shows, the overview system contains four main units, these are data processing unit, RF communication unit, sensors/meters and actuation unit and power supply management unit. The data processing unit can make valid control for other units. To have deeper look into the developed system, the block diagram of the mote functional units is shown in Fig.1.b.

The multi-sensor layer was designed to interface with number of selected sensors as well as incorporating additional capability for use within the Building environment. This includes dual actuation capabilities for any AC/DC system using an external high power relay based system for devices which consume up to 280 V and 25 A (to turn on and off appliances) as well as an onboard low power switch to enable the actuation facility. The type of on-board sensor is either digital communicating with the microcontroller through serial bus interface like I2C or analogue connected with any of the ADC channels.

The two external sensors/meters interfaces are dedicated to any meter using MODBUS protocol [8] and variable resistance temperature sensors. The MODBUS meter is exchanging data/commands through RS485 serial communications. This interface layer was also designed to incorporate external flash memory (Atmel

AT45DB041). The layer features a 4-Mbit serial flash for storing data, measurements, and remote re-programming. The photos of both the RF and sensor layers are shown in Fig.2. The complete 3 layers stackable 25mm mote is shown as well.

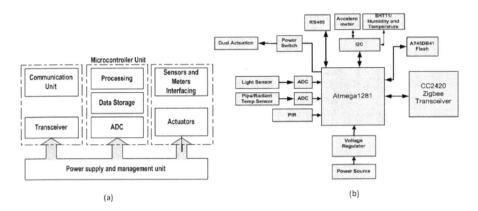

(a)   (b)

Fig. 1. (a) Top level system block diagram of the WSN mote (b) block diagram of the mote functional units

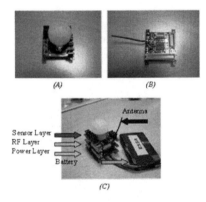

Fig. 2. Photos of the (a) Sensor layer, (b) Zigbee and processor layer, and (c) 25mm^2 mote

2.1 Sensors Selection

2.1.1 Occupation Sensor (Passive Infrared PIR)

Detecting the occupancy of the rooms inside the building was one of the essential requirements to be monitored, there was need to find suitable PIR sensor module. The Panasonic AMN44122 [9] was selected for this purpose since it provides the required functionality in a module that is smaller, more convenient and of lower energy consumption than the custom circuitry used in the prototype. Furthermore, the module provides a digital detection output that is used to trigger an interrupt on the processor when activity registers on the sensor. According to the datasheet of the PIR sensor, it has detection distance of maximum 10m (32.808ft) and detection range of 110° in horizontal and 93° in vertical.

A simple lab test has been performed to identify actual performance of the PIR sensor and obtained similar results to those in the datasheet as in Table 1. However, it was found that the actual detection region with high reliability is a little smaller than the detection region specified in the datasheet.

Table 1. The comparison of the AMN44122 PIR sensor with reference to date sheet

Items		Data Sheet	Lab test
Detection distance		10m (32.808ft)	9m (29.528ft)
Detection Range	Horizontal	110°	90°
	Vertical	93°	90°

2.1.2 Windows/Doors Status Monitoring

The detection of the windows/doors status was one of the building parameters required to be monitored by the WSN node. 3-axis accelerometer was selected for this application since it can provide useful angle information which helps to know how wide door/window is opened or closed. The LIS302DL is an ultra-compact low-power three axes linear accelerometer was integrated in the node design [10].

The main design challenge with using the accelerometer is that the microcontroller has to be continuously active to record sensor data which means high current consumption and short batter life time. In order to overcome this problem, a mechanical vibration sensor with very small package was used in this design to provide an external interrupt to the Atmel microcontroller when there is any kind of motion at any direction as presented by Fig.3.

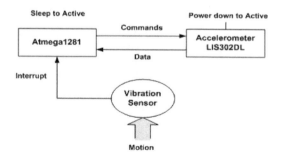

Fig. 3. Functional lock diagram of the motion sensor design

2.1.3 Water Flow /Electricity Meter Interfacing Using Modbus Handshaking

It is required to get the flow rate measurements from different locations inside the building where pipes made from different materials and have wide scale diameter size. The ultrasonic non-introductive was found to be the optimal solution for measuring the water flow rate of the water on building pipes since it is not disturbing the existing pipes installation and gives flexible testing option.   Half duplex RS485/RS232 IC was used to interface the water flow meter with the Universal Asynchronous Receiver Transmitter (UART) of microcontroller using the standard industrial MODBUS protocol [8]. The STUF-300EB flow meter from Shenitech [11] was used for this application. It provides excellent capabilities for accurate liquid flow measurement from outside of a pipe.

2.1.4 Water Pipe/Radiant Temperature Sensor Interfacing

The monitoring of the water temperature that is passing in the building pipes was needed as part of the wireless sensor system. Surface Mount Temperature Sensor from SIEMENS [12] was selected for this application as non-introductive units and can be mounted directly on a pipe inlet to sense the temperature of water passing through. The sensor performance was compared with the existing wired sensors read by the Building Management System (BMS) as shown in Table 2.

Table 2. Verifying the readings of the sensor with the existence BMS

Temp °C (BMS)	Temp °C (Sensor)	Temp °C (Calibrated Sensor)
20.25	19.01	20.01
23.12	21.03	22.03
30.45	29.5	30.5
45.21	43.2	44.2
48.87	47.62	48.62

3 Adopted Wireless Sensor Network (WSN)

3.1 WSN System Architecture

The adopted WSN architecture is based on recently released IETF IPv6 over Low power WPAN (6LoWPAN) (RFC 4944) open standard for IP communication over low-power radio devices – IEEE 802.15.4 represents one such link. WSN LoWPAN networks are connected to other IP networks through one or more border routers forwarding packets between different media including Ethernet, Wi-Fi or GPRS as shown in as shown in Fig.5 [7].

3.2 ERI Data Storage and Representation

To provide sensed data to the end user (or other software components) for the purpose of building performance monitoring (BPM), there are a number of conceptual and practical challenges that need to be overcome. The conceptual challenges can be the definition of BPM to different stakeholders of a building [13].Practical challenges include data quality, availability and consistency, and benchmarking. A Data Warehouse (DW) implementation was created to store large data sets of data provided

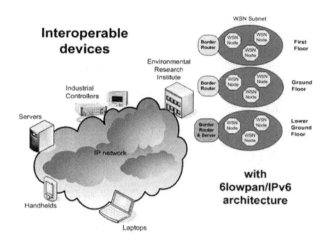

Fig. 5. WSN in the broader view

by the data streams of the WSN in ERI [14]. In Fig.6, the staging area was designed to support data from multiple sensor, meter and actuator types. This data is processed to form data cubes that support the presentation of relevant building performance measures to stakeholders.

To extract the environment information from the WSN deployment in the ERI, a Service Orientated Architecture (SOA) was used [15]. For the ERI deployment, data is gathered from the first and ground floor and sent through the wireless backbone to the embedded PC (gateway) in the basement of the building. From embedded PC, a SOA connection is maintained to a data warehouse (DW). Fig.6 shows the architecture used to gather data from the sensors and present data through a graphical user interface (GUI) to the end user.

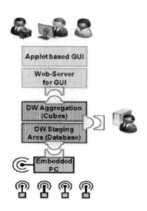

Fig. 6. SOA for WSN to DW and DW to GUI

Sample of the obtained results using a building operator GUI are displayed in Fig.7 showing one day data from light (immunology), radiant (immunology), door (seminar room) and occupancy (seminar room). Fig.8 shows samples of the selected deployment sites. In total (60) nodes were deployed in the selected three main zones within the ERI building to perform various functions of sensing and monitoring. This building performance data will be used to support decision making for facility manager and building operators to optimize maintenance activities [15] and assist in fault detection and diagnosis.

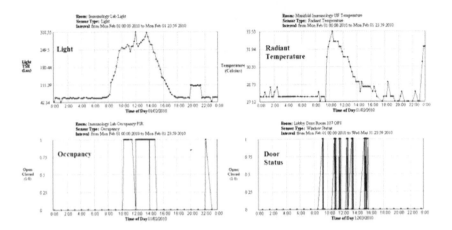

Fig. 7. GUI one day recorded data of (a) light, (b) radiant temperature, (C) occupancy and (D) Door status

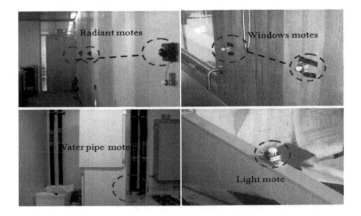

Fig. 8. Number of Deployment Sites for (Window, Radiant, Light and Water pipe)

4 Conclusions

This paper presents the design and development of a miniaturized WSN mote based on Zigbee technology for building monitoring, exploring its system control management and technology characters. The stackable technique was adopted in this work to manufacture efficiently the mote layers within small cubic size. The node can implement wide scale of stable sensors/meters data acquisition to provide the needed functions. An efficient BPM was developed to maintain the data streams from all wireless sensors to the data warehouse and at the same time provide the end user with useful information. The experiments in this paper demonstrate the capabilities and reliability of the proposed mote platform and adopted WSN topology to perform the desired tasks and extend the current BMS sensing parameters.

References

1. Gutiérrez, J.A.: Int. J. Wireless Information Networks 14, 295–301 (2007)
2. Österlind, F., Pramsten, E., Roberthson, D., Eriksson, J., Finne, N., Voigt, T.: In: Proc. IEEE Sym. On Emerging Technologies and Factory Automation, pp. 1376–1379 (2007)
3. Keller, M., O'Donnell, J., Keane, M., Menzel, K., Barton, J., Ó'Mathúna, C., Klepal, K., Pesch, D.: Buildwise: Building a Sustainable Future, Wireless Sensor Networks for Energy and Environment Management in Buildings, D1 Specification Report University College Cork (2007)
4. Jang, W.S., Healy, W.M., Skibniewski, M.J.: J. Automation in Construction 17, 729–736 (2008)
5. Reinisch, C., Kastner, W., Neugschwandtner, G., Granzer, W.: Proc. IEEE Int. Conf. on Industrial Informatics, INDIN (2007)
6. Xu, J., You, B., Cui, J., Ma, J., Li, X.: Proc. SPIE – 5th Int. Sym. on Instrumentation Science and Technology, p. 7133 (2009)
7. Spinar, R., et al.: Management with IP-based Wireless Sensor Network. In: European Wireless Sensor Networks, EWSN 2009 (2009)
8. MODBUS Industrial Protocol, http://www.modbus.org
9. AMN44122 Passive Infrared (PIR) Motion Sensor, Passive, http://pewa.panasonic.com/
10. LIS302DL, 3-axis smart digital output accelerometer, http://www.st.com
11. STUF-300EB Ultrasonic Water Flowmeter, from Shenitech, http://www.shenitech.com
12. Surface mount pipes temperature sensor, http://www.buildingtechnologies.siemens.com
13. Wang, Y., Stack, P., Tumwesigye, E., Menzel, K.: Aspects of Interface Design for Energy Management in Buildings. In: von Both, P., Koch, V. (eds.) Proc. Forum Bauinformatik, pp. 359–370. University Karlsruhe, Karlsruhe (2009); ISBN 978-3-86644-396-9
14. Ahmed, A., Menzel, K., Ploennigs, J., Cahill, B.: Aspects of Multi-dimensional Building Performance Data Management. In: Wofganghuhnt (ed.) Proc.Computing in Civil Engineering EG-ICE Conf. Computation in Civil Engineering, TU Berlin, Germany, pp. 9–16 (2009); ISBN 978-3-8322-8287-5
15. Stack, P., Manzoor, F., Cahill, B., Menzel, K.: A Service Oriented Architecture (SOA) for Building Performance Monitoring. In: Gürlebeck, K., Könke, C. (eds.) Int. Conf. on Applications of Computer Science and Mathematics in Architecture and Civil Engineering (2009)

Design and Evaluation of a Fall Detection Algorithm on Mobile Phone Platform

Manuel Silva, Pedro M. Teixeira, Filipe Abrantes, and Filipe Sousa

Fraunhofer Portugal AICOS
Rua do Campo Alegre 1021
4169-007 Porto, Portugal
{manuel.silva,pedro.teixeira,filipe.abrantes,filipe.sousa}@fraunhofer.pt

Abstract. The increasingly aging population will pose a severe burden to the health services. Falls are a major health risk that diminishes the quality of life among the elderly people and increases the health services cost. Reliable fall detection and notification is essential to improve the post-fall medical outcome which is largely dependent upon the response and rescue time. In this paper, we analyze mobile phones as a platform for developing a fall detection system. The feasibility of such platform is assessed by running an acceleration based fall detection algorithm on the phone. The algorithm was implemented for the Android OS and tested on several HTC models, which included a MEMS accelerometer. Extensive simulations of fall events as well as activities of daily life were conducted on a lab environment to evaluate the system performance. Experimental results of our system, which we still consider as work in progress, are encouraging making us optimistic regarding the feasibility of a highly reliable phone-based fall detector.

Keywords: Fall-detection, Algorithm, Accelerometer, Activities of Daily Living.

1 Introduction

Falls are dangerous, prevalent and costly. The frequency of falling is considerably higher among elderly. Nearly one third of the people aged over 65 fall every year [1]. Approximately 3% of all fallers lie for more than 20 minutes without external support [2]. The need of assistance in the case of unconsciousness or extreme injury are the main reasons why elders leave the comfort and privacy of their own home to live in an assisted-care environment (40 % of nursing home admissions are due to falls [3]). According to the world population prospects by the United Nations, the median age of the population rose from 23.9 in 1950 to 28.1 in 2005, and is forecast to rise to 37.8 by 2050 [4]. This will pose a severe burden to the health services. The financial exertion and physical requirements necessary to provide the current level of care to such a large forecast population are far too great to be feasible. Various ideas need to be produced to provide an appropriate level of care in a more efficient manner by taking advantage

S. Gabrielli, D. Elias, and K. Kahol (Eds.): AMBI-SYS 2011, LNICST 70, pp. 28–35, 2011.

of current technologies. Reliable fall detection and notification is essential in independent living facilities and in ambulatory systems for elders or patients. The objective is to improve the medical outcome which is largely dependent upon the response and rescue time. Immediate reporting to caregivers after fall event detection can certainly improve the health outcome due to faster caregiver response and appropriate medical care.

1.1   Why a Mobile Phone

Recently, technical advances in Micro Electro Mechanical System (MEMS) sensors, microprocessors and wireless communication technologies have been the driving factors to facilitate telemonitoring of people's physical activities [5]. Smaller in size, lighter in weight and relatively low cost, sensors are designed into a kind of body-attached or wearable system. The sensors collect kinetic parameters of human body and analyze data to monitor the physical activities without disturbing the wearer's daily life. A typical fall detection system has two major functional components: the fall detection component (used by the user) and the help communication component (installed indoors). The maximum distance between the sensor and the communication base is limited. Utilizing mobile phones as a fall detection system combines the detection and communication components as they present a mature hardware and software environment. They are more convenient and highly portable, enabling an outdoor fall detection system. The only prerequisite is the presence of an accelerometer to sense the user's activity. The popularity of mobile phones is likely to continuously increase in the near future due to decreasing prices, thus projecting an overall acceptance regarding it as a fall detection platform.

1.2   Major Differences When Doing It on a Mobile Phone

Carrying a mobile phone implies the user choice of its place. This in turn increases the difficulty of fall detection. The sensor location on the body relatively to the point of impact modifies the pattern of the recorded acceleration signal [6]. Besides position variability, some chaotic environments like a loose pocket might increase the turbulence of the mobile phone sensor. Another problem is the lack of a fixed referential for simpler approaches such as tilt analysis. Under static conditions a three axis accelerometer can be used to find the direction of the gravity vector, which can be used to find the tilt angle of a person relative to the gravity vector. Unfortunately, human movements are far from being static and even small motions can cause high accelerometer readings. For this reason, they are only really good for gross measurements like the analysis of intense acceleration magnitudes due to fall impacts.

1.3   Objectives

The objective of our work is threefold. Firstly, we aim at assessing the feasibility of a fall detector on a mobile phone. Is the processing speed of such devices sufficient to run the algorithm? Do the public APIs of the device grant us with the required functionality? Secondly, we want to have an idea of the order of magnitude of the accuracy that one might achieve with a phone-based fall detector. Typically, dedicated-hardware fall-detectors are positioned and fixed in certain parts of the body whereas a mobile phone is handled freely by its user and its position in the body is unknown to the fall detection application. Finally, this work has the objective of understanding the difficulties and limitations of developing a mass-market fall detection application for real handsets. Different devices will have different characteristics, from CPU speed to accelerometer accuracy. This initial approach give us a insight on the barriers one will have to overcome to achieve this goal.

1.4   Structure

The paper is organized as follows: Section 2 presents related work in the field of fall detection. In Section 3 we describe the implementation of our fall detection algorithm for the Android platform and in Section 4 we detail the specificity and sensitivity results achieved in the lab. Finally, in Section 5 we conclude the paper.

2   State of the Art and Related Work

In the past 15-20 years there have been many commercial solutions and academic developments aimed at detecting falls. The most simple and popular solutions are community alarm systems (e.g. Vivatec's Wrist Care [9]) which are based on alarm buttons located on a wrist watch or fixed in a stationary location. The main problem with those solutions is that the button is often unreachable after the fall specially when the person is unconscious [10].

Lindemann [11] created a fall detector system based on accelerometers placed into a hearing-aid housing fixed behind the ears. The sensitivity of the fall detection was assessed by acceleration patterns of the head.

The human horizontal and vertical velocity were found to be discriminatory parameters used to distinguish fall movements from normal activities [7]. During the descending phase of the fall, usually about 300 - 400 ms before the fall impact on the ground, a threshold of 1.0 ms^{-1} was identified experimentally. However it has been argued by Bourke [8] that thresholding of the vertical velocity of the trunk alone, is sufficient for fall detection, found experimentally as 1.3 ms^{-1} with 100% sensitivity and 100% specificity.

Zhang [12] placed a tri-axial accelerometer in a mobile-phone, and monitored the following sequence of events: a daily activity, fall and then person remaining motionless. In [13] was also proposed a pervasive fall detection system implemented on mobile phones.

Besides wearable sensors, image processing of video signals can also be used to detect a fall by either identifying the lying posture using scene analysis or by detecting abrupt movements. While these techniques are well established in controlled environments (laboratory, scene), they must be modified in uncontrolled environments where one controls neither the lighting nor the framing [14]. These techniques are becoming feasible, both technically and financially, thanks to the emergence of low cost cameras (web cams), the possibility to wirelessly transmit images over short distances and the availability of the required algorithms. Nevertheless the acceptance of this technology poses a major problem, as it requires the placement of video cameras in the person's living space, and in particular in the bedroom and the bathroom, with consequent concerns of privacy.

3   Mobile Phone Fall Detection

Detecting user falls on a mobile phone is significantly more difficult than doing so with dedicated fixed equipment. The mobile phone is handled freely by the user, therefore the sensor orientation is also variable, invalidating its analysis for the purpose of user position. Besides this, the MEMS accelerometer technology embedded in current mobile phones has limited accuracy and suffers from value drifting depending on the phone orientation. Finally, if one aims at developing a truly global solution, one that works across different mobile phone models, or even different operating systems, there is one extra layer of complexity that needs to be handled. Different phones will have different hardware specifications and operating system configurations, thus fall detection algorithms running on different phone models will have to deal with accelerometer data with variable precision and polling frequency. Before any data analysis can be carried out by the algorithm, it is crucial that all these effects are taken into account and that the data is normalized to the reference implementation.

3.1   The Algorithm

The fall detection algorithm was designed as a state machine, which is a simplified version of the algorithm proposed by [16]. The behavior model is composed by five finite states: *normal, fall, impact, recovery* and *unconscious* states as illustrated in Fig. 1. Transitions between states are done by inspecting the acceleration values and by analyzing its symbolic sequences. The states can be divided into two distinct phases, the pre-fall phase and post-fall phase.

Beginning at the *normal* state (pre-fall phase), if a "free-fall" acceleration profile is reached by reading acceleration values below a minimum threshold, the *fall* state is reached. Once in the *fall* state, the algorithm will record the minimum reached acceleration value and an inversion of acceleration polarity with high magnitude values are monitored within a time frame to check if a person suffers an impact. If the maximum acceleration value exceeds a threshold value, the *impact* state is reached otherwise it returns to the *normal* state. Once in the *impact* state, the algorithm will check if the difference of maximum and minimum acceleration values exceeds a threshold in order to confirm the fall event or to discriminate it as an ADL (Activities of Daily Living). If the threshold is not exceeded the algorithm moves directly to the *recovery* state and enters the post-fall phase otherwise it returns to the *normal* state. During the *recovery*

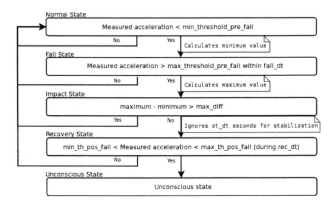

Fig. 1. Fall detection algorithm

Table 1. Threshold values and units of the different parameters for the fall-detection algorithm

Threshold	Value	Unit
min_threshold_pre_fall	8.00	m/s^2
max_threshold_pre_fall	13.42	m/s^2
max_diff	12.00	m/s^2
fall_dt	2000	ms
st_dt	7500	ms
min_th_pos_fall	9.35	m/s^2
max_th_pos_fall	10.45	m/s^2
rec_dt	5000	ms

phase it will check for user inactivity by monitoring if the acceleration values exceeds the vicinity of the passive acceleration profile value (1G) by a certain small threshold. If it does, the algorithm assumes the user has recovered from the fall and returns to the *normal* state. However, if the acceleration values do not leave the vicinity of the reference value, it is assumed that the user was unable to recover from the fall and the algorithm enters the *unconscious* state, triggering an alarm which consists in sending an SMS and Email to some pre-defined emergency contact.

The threshold values used in the fall-detection algorithm resulted from the analysis of a set of 120 recorded simulated falls and non fall activities on a lab environment and are presented in Table 1.

3.2   Implementation

The algorithm was implemented for the Android platform and tested on 5 different phone models: HTC G1, Samsung i7500, HTC Desire, HTC Desire HD and the Google Nexus 1. The fall detection function was embedded in a broader activity monitoring application called 'Mover' that is available on the Android Market. The application is composed by 3 modules:

- **Background Service** a long-standing process running in the background responsible for collecting data from the accelerometer and processing it,
- **Application User Interface** an Android activity that shows a summary of the user activity throughout the day,
- **Application Preferences** an Android preference activity that allows the user to toggle the fall-detection function as well as to configure the SMS and e-mail emergency contacts.

More interesting perhaps, are our findings regarding the accelerometer data capture on these devices. We found out that the polling frequency can vary from approximately 20 to 40 ms on the HTC models and it is never a fixed interval. On the Samsung model we were unable to reduce the accelerometer polling frequency below an average of 250 ms. Furthermore, we observed that the reference acceleration value while the phone was resting on a table would vary significantly depending on the phone orientation (horizontal versus vertical); we observed the reference acceleration value to vary between approximately 9.4 and 10.1 ms^{-2}.

4   Results of Fall Detection Algorithm

We performed the final experiment using a HTC Desire HD mobile phone running the fall detection algorithm. As the goal is to distinguish fall events from other safe daily activities, we analyzed the algorithm performance on both activities.

4.1   Evaluation Method

The algorithm performance was measured through a series of specific activity tests proposed as evaluation of fall detectors [15]. It contains 20 test scenarios for the evaluation of fall sensors, with 50% "negative" and 50% "positive" fall activities. The algorithm was tested in a laboratory environment performing falls onto a crash mat and normal activities in order to evaluate its performance. At the beginning of the trial, a mobile phone running the algorithm was placed in the pocket of each subject at the thigh position. The subjects were 10 young (<30 years) healthy males. The mean±standard deviation age, height and mass of the subjects were 26,2±3,04 years, 1,776±0,052m, and 78,3±5,3kg respectively. Each activity was performed 3 times for each subject obtaining an amount of 600 activity tests.

4.2   Data Analysis

An activity result is binary and need statistical analysis on a series of tests. There exists four possible situations:

- True positive (TP): a fall occurs and the device detects it.
- False positive (FP): the device announces a fall, but it did not occur.
- True negative (TN): a normal (no fall) movement is performed, the device does not declare a fall.
- False Negative (FN): a fall occurs but the device does not detect it.

In [15] was also proposed a classification and evaluation of fall detectors. Two criteria were proposed to evaluate the response to these four situations. Sensitivity (the capacity to detect a fall, Eq. (1)) and specificity (the ability to detect only a fall, Eq. (2)).

$$sensitivity = \frac{TP}{TP + FN} \qquad (1)$$

$$specificity = \frac{TN}{TN + FP} \qquad (2)$$

Results have shown that falls can be distinguished from normal activities with a sensitivity of 92.67% and a specificity of 72.67%. Poorer fall detection precision was achieved on falls ending on the knees (33,33% not detected) and the activity with highest amount of false positives was lying down as it was on a bed and then rising up (60% of false alarms).

5 Conclusion and Future Work

In this paper we have designed, implemented and evaluated a fall detection algorithm for mobile phones. Despite other similar experiments [13] within the past year and the fact that fall-detection has been a topic of research for almost a decade, we believe that fall-detection through a mobile phone is a research topic that is still in its infancy. We regard our work as an initial approach to the problem and our main objective with this experiment is to assess the overall feasibility of such system, both in terms of implementation on real hardware and software as well as expectable performance.

The results we have obtained are encouraging. We were able to implement a fall-detection algorithm on real hardware and observed that the processing power of current phones is more than sufficient to process the accelerometer data in real-time. At the same time the lab results showed that our algorithm was able to distinguish falls from normal activities with a sensitivity of 92.67% and a specificity of 72.67%.

Our implementation effort also provided us with insight on the practical hurdles of developing a phone-based fall detector. We learned that the accelerometer polling frequency as well as its reference values vary from model to model, something that has to be taken into account in the algorithm design.

In summary, the findings described in this paper provide us the ground for future refining of our phone-based fall detection algorithm and expect they do so also for others in the research community.

References

1. Masud, T., Morris, R.: Epidemiology of falls. Epidemiology of falls Age 30 (2001)
2. Tinetti, M.E., Doucette, J.T., Claus, E.B.: The contribution of predisposing and situational risk factors to serious fall injuries. Journal of the American Geriatrics Society 43 (1995)
3. Bezon, J., Echevarria, K.H., Smith, G.B.: Nursing outcome indicator: preventing falls for elderly people. Outcomes Management for Nursing Practice 3 (1999)
4. United Nations.: World Population Prospects. The 2004 Revision: Economic & Social Affairs (2005)
5. Aminian, K., Najafi, B.: Capturing human motion using body-fixed sensors: outdoor measurement and clinical applications. Computer Animation and Virtual Worlds 15 (2004)
6. Doughty, K., Lewis, R., McIntosh, A.: The design of a practical and reliable fall detector for community and institutional telecare. J. Telemed. Telecare (2000)
7. Wu, G.: Distinguishing fall activities from normal activities by velocity characteristics. Journal of Biomechanics 33 (2000)
8. Bourke, A.K., O'Donovan, K.J., Olaighin, G.: The identification of vertical velocity profiles using an inertial sensor to investigate pre-impact detection of falls. Med. Eng. Phys. (2008)
9. http://www.obsmedical.com/products/telecare-assisted-living/vivatec-nurse-call-system (accessed October 27, 2010)
10. Porteus, J., Brownsell, S.: Using telecare: exploring technologies for independent living for older people. Anchor Trust, Kidlington (2000)
11. Lindemann, U., Hock, A., Stuber, M., Keck, W., Becker, C.: Evaluation of a fall detector based on accelerometers: A pilot study. Medical & Biological Engineering & Computing 43 (2005)
12. Zhang, T.: Fall detection by embedding an accelerometer in cellphone and using KFD algorithm. International Journal of Computer Science and Network Security (2006)
13. Jiangpeng, D., Xiaole, B., Zhimin, Y., Zhaohui, S., Dong, X.: PerFallD: A pervasive fall detection system using mobile phones. In: 8th IEEE International Conference on Pervasive Computing and Communications Workshops, PERCOM Workshops (2010)
14. Noury, N.: Fall detection - Principles and Methods. In: 29th Annual International Conference of the IEEE Engineering in Medicine and Biology Society (2007)
15. Noury, N., Rumeau, P., Bourke, A.K., Laighin, G., Lundy, J.E.: A proposal for the classification and evaluation of fall detectors. In: IRBM, vol. 29 (2008)
16. Garret, B.: An accelerometer Based Fall Detector: Development, Experimentation, and Analysis. Report (2005)

System Performance of an LTE MIMO Downlink in Various Fading Environments

Constantinos T. Angelis and Spyridon K. Chronopoulos

Department of Informatics and Telecommunications,
Technological Educational Institute of Epirus, Arta, Greece
{kangelis,schronopoulos}@teiep.gr

Abstract. This article presents simulation results for a realistic implementation of the downlink MIMO LTE Release 8 standard in fading environments. A 4x2 MIMO Channel configuration has been used as a basis in the simulation scenarios and various key characteristics of the MIMO channel and the LTE radio interface, including physical layer and radio resource management functions ware simulated and their impact on system performance is evaluated in both local and wide area scenarios. The results suggest that in practice multi-user LTE is able to support multi stream transmission with very high data rates, even for small hand held terminals. Moreover, the improvements of 4x2 MIMO transmissions for different system configurations are clearly shown over different MIMO channel environments. In depth analysis of the individual system characteristics indicates that these performance differences are due to rather uniform contributions from a set of distinctive features.

Keywords: LTE, Performance, MIMO, OFDM, dual-codeword, fading channel, Synchronization signals.

1 Introduction

The growing demands for broadband wireless data communications, in multihop capable interfaces, are becoming more and more intense due to their improvements of coverage and capacity. For these reasons they are proposed for the next generation cellular systems like 3G-LTE [1]. This has motivated many research efforts in the last years, puts high pressure on operators to increase the capacities of their networks and on the industry for enabling such an increase also in the long term future via more efficient and flexible communication standards. Long-Term Evolution (LTE) is an emerging radio access network technology standardized in 3GPP [1], that meets all the previous constrains, and evolving as an evolution of Universal Mobile Telecommunications System (UMTS). LTE uses Orthogonal Frequency Division Multiplexing OFDM as downlink air interface multiple access scheme [1].

OFDM, which is a multi-carrier modulation scheme, uses a set of subcarriers to transmit the information symbols in parallel over the channel. One of its main advantages is increased robustness against frequency selective fading and narrowband

S. Gabrielli, D. Elias, and K. Kahol (Eds.): AMBI-SYS 2011, LNICST 70, pp. 36–43, 2011.
© Institute for Computer Sciences, Social Informatics and Telecommunications Engineering 2011

interference [2-5]. Efficient implementation of OFDM systems is based in the use of rather simple FFTs in both the transmitter and receiver. This characteristic makes such systems suitable for future high-datarate wireless systems [4-6]. Moreover the overall system reliability is increased with the use of multiple antennas in both the transmitter and receiver [7,8]. Despite these advantages, the simultaneous use of multicarrier modulations and multiple antenna systems with Spatial multiplexing and Transmit diversity schemes has a variety of challenges that still need to be validated experimentally [9].

Many researchers work on LTE systems. General LTE concept descriptions are available in [2-10]. In these papers, the focus is on key characteristics of the LTE radio interface. A set of such key characteristics are both qualitatively discussed and quantitatively evaluated in terms of downlink user data rates, spectrum efficiency generated by means of system level simulations and measurements. In [3] the performance of two dual-codeword SU-MIMO schemes, i.e. Per Antenna Rate Control (PARC) and Precoded MIMO (PREC) is studied in an OFDM deployment for LTE Release 6. In [10] some key characteristics of the LTE radio interface are compared to WiMax in 2 GHz, including physical layer and radio resource management functions, and their impact on system performance is evaluated. In [11] the principle coordination tasks of OFDMA resources in the singlehop and multihop case are discussed. In [12] downlink simulation results for a realistic implementation of the LTE standard are presented. In [13] a real implementation of a 4x4 broadband wireless MIMO-OFDM testbed based on an extension of the IEEE 802.11g/a physical layer (PHY) to multiple antenna scenarios is presented. Finally, in [14] a comparative performance analysis of the different families of solutions for the detection of Primary Synchronization Signals (P-SS) within LTE cell search procedure is proposed.

In this paper we investigate the impact of using synchronization signals (P-SS and S-SS), that are transmitted on each Tx antenna, in the FDD overall performance in both local and wide area scenarios and also for both Transmit Diversity and Open-loop Spatial Multiplexing transmission modes with 4 antennas in the transmitter and 2 antennas in the receiver. Frequency division duplex (FDD) is preferred for large area coverage and is the preferred mode for the LTE [1]. The novelty of the presented paper is the investigation of the use of synchronization signals (P-SS and S-SS) in fading environments for both in both local and wide area scenarios. These conditions mainly occur when the FDD OFDMA MIMO LTE systems are indented to be used in vehicular and urban environments, cases that are present in Ambient Assisted systems and applications. The rest of the paper is organized as follows: Section 2 describes the FDD MIMO LTE system level model; Section 3 presents an overview about the simulation model used for the investigation with description of the performed link and system level simulations; Section 4 presents the simulation results; and finally the conclusions are given in Section 5.

2   The FDD MIMO LTE Simulation Model

This section presents the simulation setup environment. The simulation results ware obtained with the Agilent Advanced Design System (ADS) [15]. We performed TDD downlink MIMO 4x2 coded measurements on fading channels for all the combinations of the parameters discussed bellow. Figure 1 shows a schematic diagram of the simulation model that consists in three main blocks: transmitter, channel and receiver chains.

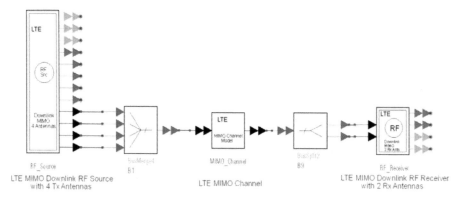

Fig. 1. The FDD MIMO LTE simulation model

Table 1. LTE System fundamental simulation conditions and parameters

Parameter	Value
Carrier Frequency	2.6 GHz
Bandwidth	5 MHz
Frame Mode	TDD Configuration
Oversampling	Ratio 2
Cyclic Prefix	Normal
Antenna Configuration	4x2
Number of code word(s)	2 for Spatial multiplexing, 1 for Transmit diversity
Number of layer(s)	2 for Spatial Multiplexing, 4 for Transmit diversity
Correlation	Low ($\alpha=0$, $\beta=0$), Medium ($\alpha=0.3$, $\beta=0.9$), High ($\alpha=0.9$, $\beta=0.9$)

The signal source follows the definition of reference channel in A.3 of TS 36.101 [1] with the exception that no Physical Hybrid ARQ Indicator Channel (HARQ) transmissions are employed and a Bandwidth of 5 MHz is employed. The modulation types that we used in our simulation scenarios are (a) 5 MHz QPSK 1/3, (b) 5 MHz 16QAM 1/2 and (c) 5 MHz 64QAM 3/4. Transmit diversity and Open-loop spatial multiplexing transmission modes were used with 4 transmitter antennas and 2 receiver antennas. Fading channels following the definition in Annex B of TS 36.101 [1]. The channel settings that were used are [1]: Extended Vehicular A model with low Doppler frequency of 5Hz (EVA 5 Hz), Extended Typical Urban model with medium Doppler frequency of 70Hz (ETU 70 Hz) and Extended Typical Urban model with high Doppler frequency of 300Hz (ETU 300 Hz). The correlation matrix support was set to Low, Medium and High. Table 1 shows some of the most fundamental simulation conditions and parameters.

In MIMO systems there is correlation between transmit and receive antennas. For maximum capacity it is desirable to minimize the correlation between transmit and receive antennas. Three different correlation levels are defined in the LTE specification TS 36.101: (i) low or no correlation (ii) medium and (iii) high correlations. The parameters α and β are defined for each level of correlation as shown in Table 1. The channel spatial correlation matrix (R_{spat}) for the 4x2 case is defined as:

$$R_{spat} = R_{eNB} \otimes R_{UE} = \begin{bmatrix} 1 & \alpha^{1/9} & \alpha^{4/9} & \alpha \\ \alpha^{1/9^*} & 1 & \alpha^{1/9} & \alpha^{4/9} \\ \alpha^{4/9^*} & \alpha^{1/9^*} & 1 & \alpha^{1/9} \\ \alpha^* & \alpha^{4/9^*} & \alpha^{1/9^*} & 1 \end{bmatrix} \otimes \begin{bmatrix} 1 & \beta \\ \beta^* & 1 \end{bmatrix} \tag{1}$$

where R_{eNB} and R_{UE} are the independent correlation matrices at UE and eNodeB respectively.

Primary and secondary synchronization signals are transmitted in the downlink to enable the UE to acquire time and frequency synchronization with a cell. The primary synchronization signal (P-SS) identifies the symbol timing and the cell ID within a cell ID group, while the secondary synchronization signal (S-SS) identifies the cell ID group. The Primary and Secondary Synchronization Signals (P-SS/S-SS) are transmitted on all the transmit antenna ports. In LTE, 3 different P-SS are generated from a frequency domain Zadoff-Chu sequence, according to [1, 14, 16, 17]:

$$d_\mu(n) = \begin{cases} \exp\left(-j\dfrac{\pi\mu(n+1)}{63}\right) & n = 0,1,....30 \\ \exp\left(-j\dfrac{\pi\mu(n+1)(n+2)}{63}\right) & n = 31,32,....61 \end{cases} \tag{2}$$

where $d_\mu(n)$ denotes the P-SS and μ denotes the sequence root index, which is 25, 29, or 34.

Cell search procedure is an essential process that allows a mobile terminal to acquire time and frequency parameters and thereafter be able to demodulate downlink and/or to transmit uplink data. In LTE, this procedure is mainly realized through the broadcast of Primary Synchronization Signal (P-SS) and Secondary Synchronization Signal (S-SS). The Primary Synchronization Signals (P-SS) are used for the identification of the physical layer cell identity, while the Secondary Synchronization Signals (S-SS) are used for the identification of the physical layer cell identity group. Thus, knowledge of the P-SS and S-SS impact in the overall LTE Performance is helpful in alleviating the detection problems.

3   Results and Discussion

Performance of the simulated schemes is compared in terms of Tx and Rx Signal Spectrum, Complementary Cumulative Distribution Function (CCDF), BER and FER measurements. Simulations were made for both presence and absence of synchronization signals (P-SS/S-SS), which in the former case were used according to [14]. The Real and Imaginary part of the FDD Downlink LTE waveforms in the 4 transmit antennas that we used are shown in figure 2. For simplicity 1 Slot is shown. Figure 3 presents indicative Signal spectrums in the 4 transmit antennas and in the 2 receive antennas for E_b / N_o = 20dB. The modulation scheme in figures 2 and 3 is QPSK 1/3, while the correlation was set to medium.

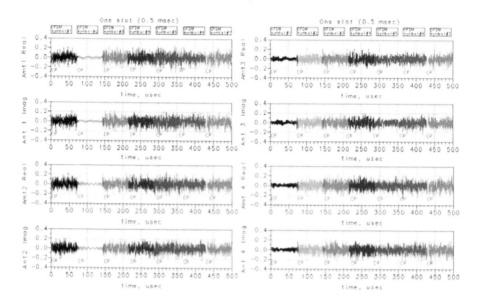

Fig. 2. Real and Imaginary part of the FDD Downlink LTE waveforms in the 4 transmit antennas

Fig. 4 shows Complementary Cumulative Distribution Function (CCDF) measurements of the TDD Downlink LTE signals in the 2 receive (Rx) antennas for (a) Spatial multiplexing and (b) Transmit diversity MIMO Mode for $E_b / N_o = 20dB$, medium correlation and for different MIMO channel models [1]: Extended Vehicular A model with low Doppler frequency of 5Hz (EVA 5 Hz), Extended Typical Urban model with medium Doppler frequency of 70Hz (ETU 70 Hz) and Extended Typical Urban model with high Doppler frequency of 300Hz (ETU 300 Hz). The modulation scheme is QPSK 1/3.

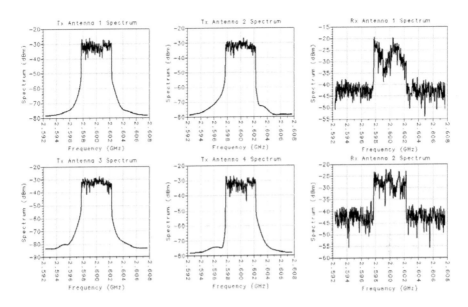

Fig. 3. Signal spectrums in the 4 transmit (Tx) antennas and in the 2 receive (Rx) antennas for E_b / N_o = 20dB

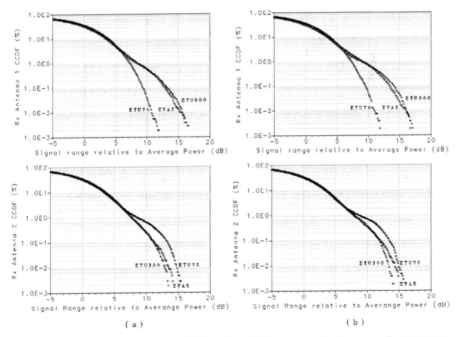

Fig. 4. CCDF measurements of the TDD Downlink LTE signals in the 2 receive (Rx) antennas for (a) Spatial multiplexing and (b) Transmit diversity MIMO Mode for E_b / N_o = 20dB

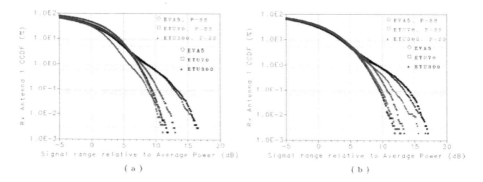

Fig. 5. CCDF measurements in different environments (EVA5, ETU70, ETU300) in the first receive (Rx) antenna for (a) Spatial multiplexing and (b) Transmit diversity MIMO Mode, with or without P-SS signals

Fig. 5 shows Complementary Cumulative Distribution Function (CCDF) measurements of the TDD Downlink LTE signals in the first receive (Rx) antenna for (a) Spatial multiplexing and (b) Transmit diversity MIMO Mode for $E_b / N_o = 20dB$, medium correlation and for different MIMO channel models [1]: (EVA 5 Hz), (ETU 70 Hz) and (ETU 300 Hz), when P-SS signals are transmitted or not. The modulation scheme is QPSK 1/3. As it is clearly seen, the use of P-SS signals affects the CCDF in the case of (EVA 5 Hz) and (ETU 300 Hz), while in the case of (ETU 70 Hz) the use of P-SS signals practically does not affect the CCDF. These results are in accordance with [4], where the WiMax IEEE 802.16-2005 system is studied.

4   Conclusion

In this paper the impact of using synchronization signals, that are transmitted on each Tx antenna, in the FDD overall performance in both local and wide area scenarios and also for both Transmit Diversity and Open-loop Spatial Multiplexing transmission modes with 4 antennas in the transmitter and 2 antennas in the receiver was investigated. Results show that, when QPSK 1/3 is used as modulation scheme, the use of P-SS signals affects the overall system performance when they are used in the case of Extended Vehicular A model with low Doppler frequency of 5Hz (EVA 5 Hz) and Extended Typical Urban model with high Doppler frequency of 300Hz (ETU 300 Hz), while in the case of Extended Typical Urban model with medium Doppler frequency of 70Hz (ETU 70 Hz) the use of P-SS signals practically does not affect the CCDF.

Acknowledgments. The Authors would like to thank Agilent, Inc. for the license to use ADS for educational and research purposes.

References

1. TS 36.101 3rd Generation Partnership Project; Technical Specification Group Radio Access Network; Evolved Universal Terrestrial Radio Access (E-UTRA); User Equipment (UE) radio transmission and reception (Release 8)
2. Hara, S., Prasad, R.: Multicarrier Techniques for 4G Mobile Communications, 27–98 (2003)
3. Virtej, E., Kuusela, M., Tuomaala, E.: System Performance of Single-User MIMO in LTE Downlink. In: IEEE International Symposium on Personal, Indoor and Mobile Radio Communications 2008 (PIMRC 2008), Cannes, September 15-18 (2008)
4. Koliopanos, C., Chronopoulos, S., Tzechilidou, A., Angelis, C.T.: Simulation, Modeling, and Performance Analysis of IEEE 802.16e OFDMA Systems for Urban and Rural Environments. In: International Conference on Signals, Circuits & Systems (SCS 2008), Tunisia, November 7-9 (2008)
5. Angelis, C.T., Koliopanos, C., Chronopoulos, S.: UWB MB-OFDM outdoor signal propagation in the presence of mobile WiMax interferers. In: Proceedings of Workshop on Next Generation Mobile Networks, WNGMN 2009, Tangiers, Morocco, November 15-17 (2009)
6. Bingham, J.A.C.: Multicarrier modulation for data transmission: an idea whose time has come. IEEE Communications Magazine 28(5), 5–14 (1990)
7. Foschini, G.J., Gans, M.J.: On limits of wireless communications in a fading environment when using multiple transmit antennas. Wireless Personal Communications (6), 311–335 (1998)
8. Zheng, L., Tse, D.N.C.: Diversity and multiplexing: a fundamental tradeoff in multiple-antenna channels. IEEE Transactions on Information Theory 49(5), 1073–1096 (2003)
9. Sampath, H., Talwar, S., Tellado, J., Erceg, V., Paulraj, A.: A fourth-generation MIMO-OFDM broadband wireless system: design, performance, and field trial results. IEEE Communications Magazine 40(9), 143–149 (2002)
10. Furuskar, A., Jonsson, T., Lundevall, M.: The LTE Radio Interface – Key Characteristics and Performance. In: IEEE International Symposium on Personal, Indoor and Mobile Radio Communications 2008 (PIMRC 2008), Cannes, September 15-18 (2008)
11. Schoenen, R., Eichinger, J., Walke, B.H.: On OFDMA FDD mode in 3G- LTE. In: 12th International OFDM-Workshop 2007 (InOWo 2007), Hamburg, Germany, August 29-30 (2007)
12. Yngve, S., Asplund, H.: 3G LTE Simulations Using Measured MIMO Channels. In: IEEE Global Telecommunications Conference (GLOBECOM 2008), New Orleans, LO, November 30- December 4 (2008)
13. Nieto, X., Ventura, L., Mollfulleda, A.: GEDOMIS: A Broadband Wireless MIMO-OFDM Testbed. Design and Implementation. In: 2nd International IEEE/Create-Net Conference on Testbeds and Research Infrastructures for the Development of Networks and Communities (TRIDENTCOM 2006), Barcelona, Spain, March 1- 3 (2006)
14. Mazarico, J.I., Capdevielle, V., Feki, A., Kumar, V.: In: LTE networks, 2nd IFIP Wireless Days (WD), Paris, France, December 15-17 (2009)
15. Agilent Advanced Design System (ADS), http://www.agilent.com
16. Sesia, S., Baker, M., Toufik, I.: LTE, The UMTS Long Term Evolution: From Theory to Practice, pp. 141–149. John Wiley & Sons, Chichester (2009)
17. Dahlman, E., Parkvall, S., Skold, J., Beming, P.: 3G Evolution: HSPA and LTE for Mobile Broadband. Elsevier, Amsterdam (2007)

Development of Computer Vision Algorithm for Surgical Skill Assessment

Gazi Islam[1], Kanav Kahol[1], John Ferrara[2], and Richard Gray[3]

[1] Dept. of Biomedical Informatics, Arizona State University, Phoenix, AZ 85004
[2] Phoenix Integrated Surgical Residency, Phoenix, AZ 85006
[3] Department of Surgery, Mayo Clinic, Scottsdale, AZ 85054
{gislam,kanav}@asu.edu, johnj@ferrara.cc, gray.richard@mayo.edu

Abstract. Advances in medical field have introduced new and progressive ways to intensify surgical resident training and surgical skills learning by developing systematic simulator training programs alongside traditional training. Both training methods need constant presence of a competent surgeon to subjectively assess the surgical dexterity of the trainee. Several studies have been done to measure user's skill objectively and quantitatively, but all use sensors which could interfere with skill execution. Also the sterilization process in an actual surgery makes the use of sensors impossible. This paper proposes a novel video-based approach for observing surgeon's hand and surgical tool movements in both surgical operation and training. Data is captured by video camera and then explored using computer vision algorithm. Finally by analyzing basic statistical parameters, observer-independent model has been developed through objective and quantitative measurement of surgical skills.

Keywords: Skill Assessment, Surgical Training, Computer Vision, Motion Tracking.

1 Introduction

In last few decades, as the health care delivery is faced with demands for greater accountability and patient safety, the effective surgical performance measurement has gained an increasingly high profile. Development and advances in medical field have made the surgical skill acquisition more challenging than ever. To ensure the best surgical performance, systematic simulator training programs are being developed alongside traditional training in hospitals. It has been a new and progressive way to intensify surgical resident training and surgical skills learning. The traditional training method needs constant presence of a competent surgeon for measure the progress of the trainee. The assessment is done to evaluate the surgical dexterity, is highly subjective and lacking the quantitative data [1]. Simulator-based training has become very popular as it does not involve risk and patient discomfort. Several researches have been done to address the issue of evaluating the user's performance in the simulator-based training system. For accurately measure user's skill objectively and quantitatively, the system must satisfy the following requirements [2]: (1) the system

S. Gabrielli, D. Elias, and K. Kahol (Eds.): AMBI-SYS 2011, LNICST 70, pp. 44–51, 2011.

must possess adequate sensing techniques to monitor the user's operation; (2) the system must extract relevant features from the sensing data; and (3) the system needs a good computational model to represent the skill demonstrated in the operation. Such a model is essential for accurately measuring the technical competence of the performance.

Tracking hand and surgical tool movement is one of the most important features in assessing surgical performance. Many sensor-based systems have been developed for accurate tracking of surgeon's hand or surgical tool movement. However, the integration of sensors often causes interference with the surgical execution. Moreover in actual surgery it is very difficult to use sensors as they need to be sterile. Also the extensive use of sensors makes the entire surgery and the training procedure more expensive.

This paper proposes a novel video-based approach for observing continuous, long sequence of surgeon's hand and surgical tool movements in both surgical operation or surgical training, and then modeling and evaluating the skill demonstrated in the observation. Hand movement of entire surgical procedure is captured using inexpensive video camera. Video data of the tool movement can also be obtained for minimal invasive surgery (MIS). Both of the video data are analyzed using computer vision algorithm and then integrated to correlate with user's skill level. For modeling the surgical skill, a stochastic approach is proposed that uses simple arithmetic mean and standard deviation of the processed data. Using this technique, observer-independent models can be developed through objective and quantitative measurement of surgical skills. Because of the non-contact nature of the tracking technique, the system is free from sterile issue and there is minimal interference with the skill execution, unlike other methods that employ instrumented gloves or sensor-based surgical tools.

2   Related Work

Specialized instrumented systems with the ability to measure surgical proficiency have been proposed. Examples of such systems are the BLUE-DRAGON system, MISTVR system, LapSim, ProMIS system, ROVIMAS system, WKS system, WB system, BSN technology, Immersion Simulators, etc. Many of these systems use time as a metric for measurement of surgical proficiency. Other measures of proficiency include kinematics of the laparoscopic tools (BLUE-DRAGON [3-5], ROVIMAS systems [1]). Some systems use generic measures such as smoothness of the movements as a measure of proficiency (ProMIS system [6]). WKS system [7-9] measures force and movement of the dummy skin in suture/ligature training system to evaluate performance. By using wireless sensor glove and body sensor network (BSN) technology [10], hand gesture data can be captured and analyzed with Hidden Markov Model (HMM) for surgical skill assessment. Several systems have been developed to measure performance in actual surgery. Wasada Bioinstrumentation (WB) system [11] uses a series of sensors to track head, arm and hand movement and as well as several physiological parameters to analyze surgeon's performance during laparoscopic surgery. Sadahiro, T et al. used force platform to measure fluctuations of operator's center of pressure (COP) [12] to estimate the skill level in the operating room. Most of these systems need multiple wearable sensors, which could interfere in operator's skill execution. Also the sensors need to sterile to be used in actual surgery and can make the entire surgery very expensive.

Chen, J. et al proposed a video-based system to track special markers on the glove [2]. However it requires consistent lighting and direct line-of-sight to the markers which might not be possible during actual surgery.

3 The Proposed Approach

3.1 Data Capture Setup

20 residents from different PGYN-levels have done the peg transfer exercise on Fundamental of Laparoscopic Surgery (FLS) [13] wearing purple colored gloves. Two video cameras were steadily used to capture video data of the hand movement. The internal videos from the FLS have also been recorded for capturing the tool movement.

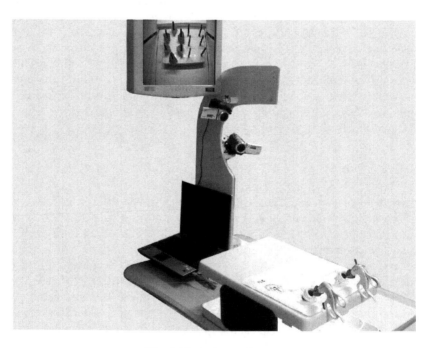

Fig. 1. Experimental setup

3.2 Methodology

Every participant has been asked to wear purple-colored surgical gloves. This color has been particularly chosen for easier detection of glove from the background objects. Then the participants chose two laparoscopic graspers and performed the pegboard transfer exercise on the FLS. The protocol for the exercise is – "Grasp a colored object with the non-dominant hand, transfer to the dominant hand and place it on the opposite side of the board. Repeat until all six have been transferred. Reverse process until initial state achieved."[13] During the exercise, hand movement has been captured using both the video cameras. Also the internal FLS video that captures tool movement has been written to the disk.

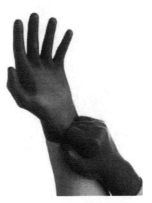

Fig. 2. Purple surgical gloves

All these video data have been analyzed by 'compute vision' algorithms [14]. In the late 1950s/early 1960s a new approach to the study of vision emerged in the form of 'compute vision'. Since then it's a rapidly developing technology that extracts and use information present in visual images. The potential practical benefits of computer vision systems are immense. The advancement of computer vision makes it very popular in the field of medical image analysis, human computer interaction (HCI), industrial inspection, security scanning, military intelligence, etc. in this paper computer vision has been applied in two steps –

1) <u>Glove/object detection:</u> Hand and tool movement videos have been analyzed using Open Source Computer Vision (OpenCV) [14] programs. The program uses histogram matching algorithm and quite accurately detects the purple gloves from the hand movement video and blue/pink colored objects from the tool movement video (Figure 5). Glove and tool detection are important as it reduces the noise that comes from other background movement captured in the video.

2) <u>Motion capture:</u> Once the glove/object detection is done, another OpenCV [14] program is used to capture movement data. The algorithm uses motion segmentation to show how an image changes over time. The trail of hand and object movement observation is done and pixel data for every frame are captured to analyze smoothness of movement (Figure 6).

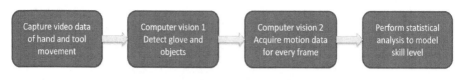

Fig. 3. Methodology

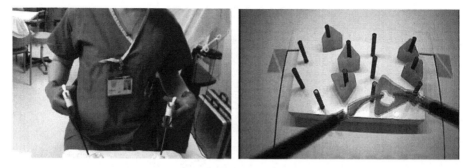

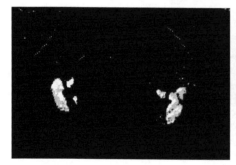

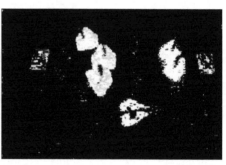

Fig. 4a. Hand movement capture   **Fig. 4b.** Tool movement capture

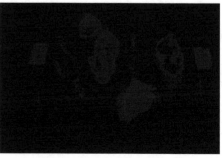

Fig. 5a. Glove detection   **Fig. 5b.** Colored object detection

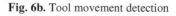

Fig. 6a. Hand movement detection   **Fig. 6b.** Tool movement detection

3.3 Data Analysis

The number of pixel value per frame for each participant has been studied with Matlab program for the hands and tools movement analysis. The lowest number of pixel value per frame is considered as the idle frame i.e. minimum or no motion. For every data-set, pixel values on each frame have been normalized using the corresponding idle frame. Arithmetic mean and standard deviation have been calculated for all the data sets. Finally, the ANOVE procedure [15] has been performed in SAS-a statistical analysis tool to observe the variance analysis.

4 Experimental Analysis/Results

The hand movements of 20 residents (5 experts, 5 intermediate and 10 novices) have been observed. Number of blue pixel per frame is inversely proportional to the smoothness of the hand movement. As we plot the normalized number of pixel over time, a clear distinction is observed between an expert, intermediate and novice (Figure 7). For expertise recognition, mean and standard deviation of each class of data have been calculated (Table 1).

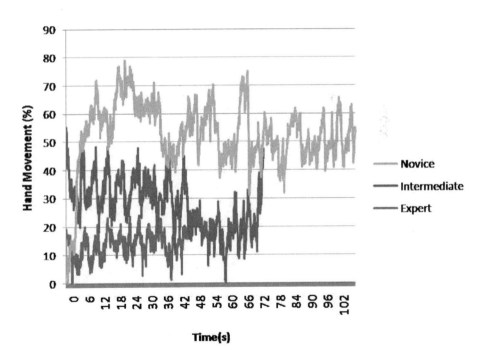

Fig. 7. Movement smoothness

Finally one-way ANOVA analysis [15] in SAS shows that the difference in mean is significant (significance probability = 0.0014). Arithmetic means with standard errors have been plotted in figure 8.

Table 1. Mean and standard deviation of data

	Expert	Intermediate	Novice
Mean	24.51	31.31	36.3
Std. Deviation	3.83	5.45	19.97

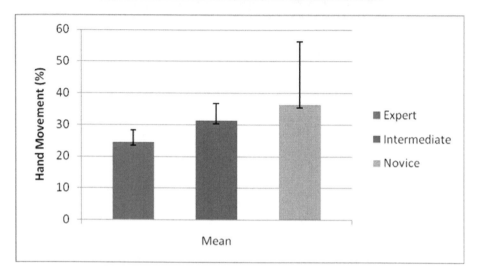

Fig. 8. ANOVA analysis

5 Conclusion and Future Work

The proposed approach indicates that computer vision based analysis of surgical movements may provide a suitable basis for expertise level analysis. Such a system will be a natural tool for evaluating surgical residents. As the system is based on the video data analysis of hand and tool movement rather than sensor-based data, it can easily be extended to provide real-time feedback to surgical interns while doing surgical exercise or to surgeons while performing an actual surgery. In, future we intend to extensively test the proposed methodology through controlled studies. Longitudinal studies will be conducted to evaluate surgical proficiency at various stages of training to fully evaluate the methodology and plot the learning curves.

References

[1] Dosis, A., Bello, F., Rockall, T., Munz, Y., Moorthy, K., Martin, S., Darzi, A.: ROVIMAS: a software package for assessing surgical skills using the da Vinci telemanipulator system. In: 4th International IEEE EMBS Special Topic Conference on Presented at Information Technology Applications in Biomedicine (2003)
[2] Chen, J.Y., Sharma, R.: Visual modelling and evaluation of surgical skill. Pattern Anal. Applic. 6, 1–11 (2003)

[3] Rosen, J., Brown, J.D., Chang, L., Sinanan, M.N., Hannaford, B.: Generalized approach for modeling minimally invasive surgery as a stochastic process using a discrete Markov model. IEEE Transactions on Biomedical Engineering 53, 399–413 (2006)

[4] Rosen, J., Brown, J.D., Chang, L., Barreca, M., Sinanan, M., Hannaford, B.: The BlueDRAGON - a system for measuring the kinematics and dynamics of minimally invasive surgical tools in-vivo. In: Proceedings of IEEE International Conference on Presented at Robotics and Automation, ICRA (2002)

[5] Rosen, J., Hannaford, B., Richards, C.G., Sinanan, M.N.: Markov modeling of minimally invasive surgery based on tool/tissue interaction and force/torque signatures for evaluating surgical skills. IEEE Transactions on Biomedical Engineering 48, 579–591 (2001)

[6] The world-leading ProMIS Surgical Simulator, http://www.haptica.com/

[7] Oshima, N., Solis, J., Ishii, H., Matsuoka, N., Hatake, K., Takanishi, A.: Acquisition of quantitative data for the detailed analysis of the suture/ligature tasks with the WKS-2R. In: 6th International Special Topic Conference on presented at Information Technology Applications in Biomedicine, ITAB (2007)

[8] Solis, J., Oshima, N., Ishii, H., Matsuoka, N., Takanishi, A., Hatake, K.: Quantitative assessment of the surgical training methods with the suture/ligature training system WKS-2RII. In: IEEE International Conference on presented at Robotics and Automation, ICRA (2009)

[9] Solis, J., Oshima, N., Ishii, H., Matsuoka, N., Hatake, K., Takanishi, A.: Development of a sensor system towards the acquisition of quantitative information of the training progress of surgical skills. In: 2nd IEEE RAS & EMBS International Conference on Presented at Biomedical Robotics and Biomechatronics, BioRob (2008)

[10] King, R.C., Atallah, L., Lo, B., Guang-Zhong, Y.: Development of a Wireless Sensor Glove for Surgical Skills Assessment. IEEE Transactions on Information Technology in Biomedicine 13, 673–679 (2009)

[11] Zecca, M., Cavallo, F., Saito, M., Endo, N., Mizoguchi, Y., Sinigaglia, S., Itoh, K., Takanobu, H., Megali, G., Tonet, O., Dario, P., Pietrabissa, A., Takanishi, A.: Using the Waseda Bioinstrumentation System WB-1R to analyze Surgeon’s performance during laparoscopy - towards the development of a global performance index. In: IEEE/RSJ International Conference on Presented at Intelligent Robots and Systems, IROS (2007)

[12] Sadahiro, T., Hamazaki, M., Miyawaki, F., Yoshimitsu, K., Masamune, K.: Laparoscopic skill measurement with COP to realize a HAM Scrub Nurse Robot system. In: IEEE International Conference on Presented at Systems, Man and Cybernetics, ISIC (2007)

[13] Fundamentals of Laparoscopic Surgery...the definitive laparoscopic skills enhancement and assessment module, http://www.flsprogram.org/

[14] Bradski, G., Kaehler, A.: Learning OpenCV: Computer Vision with the OpenCV Library. Reilly Media, Inc., Sebastopol (2008)

[15] Delwiche, L.D., Slaughter, S.J.: The Little SAS Book: A Primer, 4th edn. SAS Institue, Inc., NC (2008)

Open Architecture to Raise Awareness of Energy Consumption on the Home Environment

António Rodrigues[1], Carlos Resende[1], Filipe Sousa[1], and Ana Aguiar[2]

[1] Fraunhofer Portugal AICOS,
Rua do Campo Alegre 1021, 4169-007 Porto, Portugal
{antonio.rodrigues,carlos.resende,filipe.sousa}@fraunhofer.pt
http://www.fraunhofer.pt
[2] Faculty of Engineering, University of Porto, Instituto de Telecomunicações
R. Dr. Roberto Frias s/n, 4200-465 Porto, Portugal
anaa@fe.up.pt

Abstract. The climate changes as well as the sustainability of our energy supplies present multiple challenges and require a worldwide coordinated response. Europe 2020 is a jigsaw of policies and measures binding targets for 2020 to reduce greenhouse gas emissions by 20%, ensure 20% of renewable energy sources in the EU energy mix, and the reduction of EU global primary energy use by 20%. In the longer term, new generations of technologies have to be developed via breakthroughs in research if we are to meet the greater ambition of reducing our greenhouse gas emissions by 60-80% by 2050. The reduction of the primary energy use can be accomplished with mentality awareness of the home users. By educating ourselves and those around us, our negative behaviors can be changed, creating a culture of sustainability. In order to achieve this goal, we are suggesting an open architecture with a friendly visualization interface that can be used to raise the households inhabitants awareness of their power consumption. With the proposed architecture, energy consumption data can be stored in a remote server and can be further processed in order to extract the power consumption for each electrical appliance, opening the door to the development of service extensions to provide user- and context-aware advice on how to save energy.

Keywords: Architecture, Energy, Wireless, Sensor Network, Power, Measurement.

1 Introduction

Recently, the European Union (EU) introduced the '20-20-20 goals' [1], a set of environment and energy sustainability measures targeting the year of 2020. This commitment set briefly consists in 1) reducing the greenhouse gas emissions by 20%, 2) ensuring that 20% of the consumed energy is provided by renewable sources, and also 3) reducing the EU primary energy use by 20% [1]. An approach toward the latter relies on raising the awareness to the problem within the home, since residential energy consumption can represent 30% to

S. Gabrielli, D. Elias, and K. Kahol (Eds.): AMBI-SYS 2011, LNICST 70, pp. 52–59, 2011.

40% of the total energy demand in developed nations [2]. Studies conducted in different countries concluded that 26% to 36% of home energy consumption is a result of residents' behavior [3], giving emphasis to the importance of energy consumption awareness in improving residential energy efficiency. The next step is to understand how to encourage household inhabitants to adopt a sustainable behavior. Recent results show that household inhabitants install energy monitoring solutions in their homes mostly 'for saving money, maintaining a comfortable setting' [4] and that they wish real-time information on their in-home resource consumption [4,5]. However, this information alone may not be sufficient to effect behavioral changes, since general users may not know the course of action to follow upon a certain information set. A more effective approach is to provide consumers with sustainable education, supported by the numbers of their own consumption information as a continuous process [3,5], i.e., both before, during and after energy use.

This paper presents EMA (Energy Metering Application), an open architecture for a system with the potential to encourage sustainable energy usage within residential environments. EMA enables the collection and storage of energy consumption data from individual electrical appliances. Besides, this solution provides a user-friendly data visualization in a platform-independent manner, accessible from any device (laptop, smartphone, photo-frame, etc) connected to the Internet. The system is designed for easy setup, using the existing communication infrastructure of the household. Although EMA is in many aspects similar to existing solutions, we are unaware of a structured discussion on the issues relevant for the design of the different components and their integration into an architecture as the one proposed here.

The rest of the paper is organized as follows: Section 2 refers to existing energy metering techniques and architectures. In Section 3, we describe the system requirements and use cases. In Section 4 we detail the design of the EMA system including its key components. Finally, Section 5 concludes the paper and presents future work to be developed within the project's scope.

2   Related Work

Most of the houses in developed countries already have a system to measure overall electricity consumption and charge it accordingly. However, these systems are not designed so that the householders can understand and control their consumption costs, and commonly they are located outside the home. Recently, several energy metering systems oriented to help end-users understand their energy consumption patterns appeared in the market.

Energy-aware Plug and Play (EPnP) [6] proposes a network level power management for home network devices. The proposed power management is effective when a service requires the joint interaction of many devices, however the interaction information is kept within the house environment. This can be understood as an hidden cost to householders, since they are responsible for the maintenance of the server and for the security of the stored information. The architecture for a home energy saving system, HESS, is proposed in [7], which provides a real-time home energy monitoring service. Its main objective is to reduce or cut off standby power consumed by home appliances, thus providing an intelligent home energy management service. HESS uses a modular architecture, however the HESS server is a critical system component that must be maintained by the householder. The authors also do not clearly explain if the HESS clients are easily added or removed. The ecoMOD housing project [9] is an on-going design, build, and evaluation of a prototype which contains electrical power, water, temperature, and carbon dioxide sensors. The proposed architecture is complex, not easily deployed by the typical householder and also lacks an interface to give proper feedback to the users. The OWL Wireless Electricity Monitor [14] and Eco-Eye [15] are electricity metering systems which use contactless electric energy metering sensors (clips placed around appliance power cable) connected through wires to a wireless transmitter. A wireless receiver, equipped with a simple display, receives data from the transmitter and shows instantaneous and accumulated energy consumption translated into monetary cost. For both OWL [14] and Eco-Eye [15] the display can show data from only one transmitter that supports a limited number of energy sensors wired to it, and the user interaction is limited to an LCD display controlled through a set of buttons. TREE (Tendril Residential Energy Ecosystem) [16] uses a lower cost metering unit, consisting of a module to be placed between the device plug and the power outlet. TREE is very similar to the system proposed in this paper, but it is designed to be offered as a service by utilities or energy retailers, so it is closed and householders are obliged to buy the service from these companies. Plogg [17] is a complete metering system similar to TREE that provides electric energy metering devices with different wireless communication standards (such as Bluetooth and ZigBee) and sends the data to a backoffice, where it is available for visualization. Plogg offers functionalities which are similar to those provided by EMA, but does not support a device-independent energy consumption display and data is available outside the home only if a static IP address is used. Google Power Meter [18] and Microsoft Hohm [19] do not offer a complete energy metering system, as these focus on storage, processing and visualization of consumption data, offering services like the introduction of active and semi-personalized advices about good energy consumption policies.

A recent study on understanding resource consumption in the home [4] concluded that household inhabitants would like detailed real-time information of their in-home energy consumption as well as tips on how to save resources that are relevant to their situation. Although some were aware of the existence of systems similar to Plogg or TREE, these are perceived complex and requiring extensive rewiring [4]. Moreover, by storing the information in reliable infrastructure and applying data-mining techniques, there is the possibility to extract more meaningful information for the user [8].

3   Requirements and Use Cases

Our ultimate goal is to develop an electricity monitoring system for residential use that is capable of displaying electricity consumption in a way that motivates energy consumption savings on the inhabitants. The system described here is specific to monitoring electricity, but we envision a system that 1) can be easily extended to meter other types of energy, like gas, water or heating. This can be achieved by separating the metering part from the home communication among devices. It should 2) provide understandable information about the consumption of one or more home electrical appliances, calling for a home communication network that can support a large number of devices. Moreover, 3) that information should be accessible in real-time and 4) from any place. This has two consequences for system design: the energy data should be saved in a remote and centralized location located outside the home environment and it should have a device-independent interface so that it is accessible from anywhere. The system should 5) be easily deployable and 6) make use of as much as possible of the existing household infrastructure, driving us to decide for a wireless network to provide communication among the home devices and a router for gateway. Hence, electricity metering units responsible for gathering electricity consumption data from electrical appliances should be easily added to/removed from the system. Further, the network to be able to setup and manage all the electricity meters located in a home requiring only very little interaction. Finally, 7) it should have a an open and modular architecture, so that it can be easily enhanced with other features and integrated with other services.

4   System Architecture

We propose a system architecture following the previously defined requirements and design guidelines. The EMA system, depicted in Figure 1, consists of three main blocks: home, backoffice and user interface. While the first two are sets of physical components, the user interface consists of both the data visualization GUI and the physical devices that enable access to it. This separation is fundamental for a scalable architecture, making use of existent infrastructure (COTS router as gateway, Internet connection, GUI on existing devices) to avoid the necessity of home-located resources capable of constant data processing, saving the end-user unnecessary material, power consumption and maintenance costs. The system follows a service oriented architecture (SOA) where the home environment and user interface use services offered by the backoffice through Simple Object Access Protocol (SOAP) and AJAX. This modularity and use of open interfaces enable the easy integration of EMA or its components with other systems.

EMA must provide two basic functionalities: 1) the addition/removal of electricity meters from the system, and 2) gathering energy measurements in a remote server, for storage, processing and adequate visualization. The management of meters in the system (1) can be further split into construction and management of the energy meters network in the home, and the device addition/removal

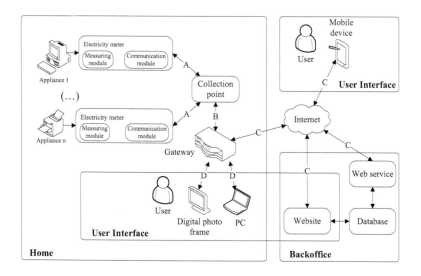

Fig. 1. EMA's system architecture

in the backoffice. The first is readily implemented by wireless technologies available in the market (e.g. ZigBee [10] or Z-Wave [11]), and is accomplished by adopting such a wireless technology for the communication between the electricity meters and the collection point. The second is achieved by running an EMA dedicated application in parallel with the other tasks normally performed by the gateway, in combination with the built-on/in collection point: the latter retrieves the list of associated electricity meters and the EMA dedicated application registers them in the remote server using an appropriate service. This process can be triggered by pushing a button on the collection point. The acquisition of an energy measurement (2) is done periodically upon a broadcast request message sent by the collection point to the electricity meters associated to the wireless sensor network. For each response sent to the collection point built-on/in the gateway, the EMA dedicated application sends the pair (meter id,measurement) to the remote backoffice server.

4.1   Electricity Meter

The electricity meter is the physical component which measures the electricity consumption of a given appliance using the Teridian 71M6511 IC [12]. The electricity meter is to be placed between the AC power outlet and the plug of the electrical appliance to be monitored, so that not only the current and voltage can be sensed, but also the power to operate collected. It contains two separate modules — measurement and communication modules — to provide a straightforward extension of the system to other types of metering, since the communication module can then be applied to any kind of energy measurement module (see requirement 1 in Section 3). The communication module consists of a wireless transceiver IC and RF front-end. We adopted the Z-Wave technology since the auto-configuration of the network and the easy addition/removal of nodes fulfills our requirements.

4.2 Gateway and Collection Point

The gateway is the point that interfaces the home environment and the Internet and the collection point is a device that serves as gateway to the network of electricity meters. It was implemented in a COTS router (specifically the Ubiquiti Routerstation Pro), a device commonly present at home and constantly turned on to provide Internet access to its users, whereas the collection point consisted of a Z-Wave USB device connected through an USB port. openWRT [13] was used as the router firmware, in order to implement the basic system functionalities described in the introductory paragraphs of Section 4. The router hosts an application that consists of two main parts, one responsible for receiving data from the collection point (via interface B) and another that sends the data to the backoffice via Internet (interface C). Again, this separation keeps the system modular: only a specific self-contained part of the application must be changed to accommodate changes in the technology used for interface B or C. Additionally, some effort was made towards the integration of EMA with the Google Power-Meter API. Besides posting the energy measurement values to a remote server these can also be easily sent to the GooglePowerMeter server and visualized in the Google Power Meter interface [18].

4.3 Backoffice

The backoffice is a server, or cluster of services, in a remote location where the energy consumption data is stored, processed and prepared for visualization. It holds a database which stores information about each user: profile, electricity meters owned, the measurements made by electricity meters over time, as well as any other statistics over those data. The communication between home and the backoffice is based on Web Services. The application running on the gateway sends SOAP requests to the backoffice that hosts a custom Web Service, exposing operations which involve interactions with the database.

4.4 User Interface

The user interacts with the system in two ways: for the installation of the meters and for visualizing the data. The first is discussed in the introductory paragraphs of Section 4. The latter is provided by the third main system block, the user interface, which groups the applications responsible for 1) processing the consumption data and 2) generating the visual information as well as 3) the renderer software. This is primarily a common browser that runs on any device with Internet access, like a mobile device or a regular PC, but it can also be an RSS feed reader on a similar device or on a photo frame, as presented in Figure 2. Alternatively, the Google PowerMeter provides both a structured platform to store energy data as well as advanced visualization functionalities [18].

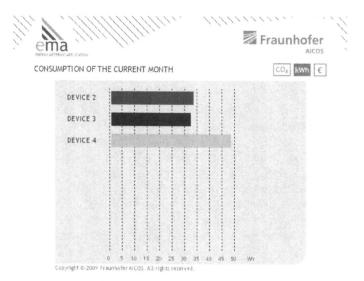

Fig. 2. EMA photo frame screenshot

5   Conclusions and Future Work

This paper presents a modular and flexible approach for detailed measurement of energy consumption in homes, offering user-friendly, platform-independent visualization of that data from any device with Internet access. The EMA architecture allowed the integration of the collection point and gateway into a router with a Z-Wave USB stick connected to it. This way the energy meter network can be easily implemented as a stand-alone system, which is deployed without the need of any type of configuration. The EMA gateway was developed taking into consideration the use cases defined in Section 3. Efforts to integrate EMA with the Google Power Meter API have been spent, despite the early stages of the developments, which allows the addition of a new visualization method and storage of the information in a reliable infrastructure. The modularity of the architecture is the key to flexible deployment of such a system, as it enables easy change/extension of any block of the system without requiring modifications to the other parts, which, in turn, enables the straightforward support of different business models for providing such a service. For future work we should focus attention in the developments of Google Power Meter API since, at the time of the development of this project, the API was still in an early stage. Additionally, the development of service extensions to provide user- and context-aware advice on how to save energy is also an issue to address. Also, other exploratory work will be done related to effective behavioral changes that can be achieved and the best means to achieve it, both in terms of information and visualization techniques and other features desired by the users. Finally, how to offer such a service in economically feasible ways remains to be discussed and studied in a systematic way.

References

1. Barroso, J.M.: 2020 by 2020: Europes Climate Change Opportunity. Speech to the European Parliament, Brussels (2008)
2. Hongbo, W., Changbin, L.: Research on Incentive Mechanism to Promote Energy Efficiency in Existing Buildings. In: IEEE International Conference on Industrial Engineering and Engineering Management, pp. 1704–1708 (2007)
3. Elias, E., et al.: Assessing User Behaviour for Changes in the Design of Energy Using Domestic Products. In: IEEE International Symposium on Electronics and the Environment, pp. 1–6 (2008)
4. Chetty, M., et al.: Getting to Green: Understanding Resource Consumption in the Home. In: Proceedings of the 10th International Conference on Ubiquitous Computing, pp. 242–251. ACM, New York (2008)
5. Ai He, H., Greenberg, S.: Motivating Sustainable Energy Consumption in the Home. In: ACM CHI Workshop on Defining the Role of HCI in the Challenges of Sustainability. ACM, New York (2009)
6. Jeong, Y., et al.: A Network Level Power Management for Home Network Devices. IEEE Transactions on Consumer Electronics 54(2), 487–493 (2008)
7. Choi, K., et al.: Architectural Design of Home Energy Saving System Based on Realtime Energy-Awareness. In: Proceedings of the 4th International Conference on Ubiquitous Information Technologies & Applications, pp. 1–5 (2009)
8. Ruzzelli, A.G., et al.: Real-Time Recognition and Profiling of Appliances through a Single Electricity Sensor. In: 7th Annual IEEE Communications Society Conference on Sensor Mesh and Ad Hoc Communications and Networks, pp. 1–9 (2010)
9. Stawitz, C.C., et al.: Increasing Awareness of Residential Energy Consumption: Data Analysis and Presentation for ecoMOD, a Sustainable Housing Initiative. In: Systems and Information Engineering Design Symposium, pp. 55–59. IEEE, Los Alamitos (2008)
10. Labiod, H., Hossam, A., De Santis, C.: Wi-Fi, Bluetooth, Zigbee and WiMax. Springer, Heidelberg (2007)
11. Walko, J.: Home Control. Computing & Control Engineering Journal 17(5), 16–19 (2006)
12. 71M6511/71M6511H, http://www.maxim-ic.com/datasheet/index.mvp/id/6845
13. OpenWRT - Wireless Freedom, http://openwrt.org/
14. 2 Save Energy Ltd., OWL Wireless Electricity Monitor, http://www.theowl.com
15. Eco-Eye Real-Time Electricity Monitor, http://aaaeco.homestead.com/index.html
16. I. Tendril Networks, Tendril - Smart Energy for Life, http://www.tendrilinc.com/
17. Plogg: Wireless Energy Management, http://www.plogginternational.com/ploggproducts.html
18. Google, Google PowerMeter, http://www.google.org/powermeter/
19. Microsoft, Microsoft Hohm, http://www.microsoft-hohm.com/default.aspx

RFID-Based System for Tracking People: Approaches to Tagging Demented Patients

Aleksandar Matic, Venet Osmani, and Oscar Mayora

CREATE-NET, Via alla Cascata 56/D, 38123 Povo, Trento, Italy
{aleksandar.matic,venet.osmani,oscar.mayora,
silvia.gabrielli}@create-net.org

Abstract. RFID technology has proven to be an effective solution in many applications for monitoring demented patients. However, its wider acceptance is still limited by prohibitive deployment costs, technological limitations and privacy concerns. In this paper, an RFID-based indoor tracking system was analyzed regarding an additional barrier of RFID's acceptance which is an issue of choosing an appropriate strategy for tagging patients. This includes making the trade-off between technological constraints, healthcare staff's routines and the fact that patients with dementia may tend to remove foreign objects.

Keywords: RFID, indoor tracking, monitoring patients, tagging patients.

1 Introduction

Rapid development of technology and medicine in the last decades allowed for significantly higher life expectancy thus shifting median age of population. These trends are predicted to occur in the future – by 2030 the predicted number of people over 65 years will be approximately 71.5 million only in the US [1]. As an inevitable consequence of this growth it is reasonable to expect an increasing number of patients suffering various diseases that are typical of old age, and as such increasing care provisioning demand. In particular, prevalence of dementia is doubling every five years in patients over age of 65 [2]. Dementia causes a deterioration of cognitive functions endangering independence and quality of life, while at the same time making it an expensive disease to monitor and treat.

Addressing the aging population needs there is an increasing body of research initiatives aiming to monitor patients with dementia by exploiting technological solutions. As computational capabilities continuously improve and sensing devices shrink in size, the use of technology is allowing monitoring many aspects of patients' life, from their activities up to various physiological parameters, while increasingly becoming more and more integrated into the living environments. The ultimate goal is development of an unobtrusive system capable of reliable operation while being cost-effective; however, typically there is a trade-off between these requirements.

Although not initially intended for monitoring demented patients, RFID (Radio Frequency Identification) technology has proved to be an effective solution for this purpose, owing to its design (differently sized and shaped tags that can be identified

S. Gabrielli, D. Elias, and K. Kahol (Eds.): AMBI-SYS 2011, LNICST 70, pp. 60–65, 2011.

without a direct line of sight from antennas) and innovative applications. Using solely RFID or combining it with other technologies, significant results are achieved in analyzing numerous activities of daily living, an important monitoring aspect for demented subjects. For instance, Wu et al [3] achieved a high recognition rate in 16 kitchen activities using RFID, Woodward Laboratories developed the system for monitoring hand hygiene [4], RFID-based design for controlling medication intake is addressed by Ho et al [5] while our previous work [6] tackles the problem of automatic monitoring of steps in dressing activity exploiting the fusion of RFID and the video machine system. With an RFID reader embedded in a glove Philipose et al. [7] recognized 14 everyday activities based on objects manipulated by subjects. Using RFID for identification and localization in addition to other sensors intended for capturing activity patterns, Kaye [8] detected trajectories of change, recorded over many years and analyzed variability in patients' behavior, aiming to dementia prevention. Relying on active RFID-based system for positioning, Kearns et al. [9] correlated patterns of subject's movements and levels of cognitive impairment. In addition, RFID technology proved to be suitable in a number of other healthcare systems, due to the possibility of quickly retrieving patient information and monitoring patient's location [10].

However, RFID implementation in healthcare applications is still behind earlier optimistic expectations of its wide acceptance and according to Yao et al. [10] major barriers lie in prohibitive deployment costs, technological limitations and privacy concerns.

The authors of this paper, in turn, identify and analyze an additional barrier of RFID's acceptance: tagging objects of interests, subjects and the fact that patients with dementia may tend to remove foreign objects. In order to track subjects, we have designed a RFID-based system that is able to track transitions between rooms of interest and we have evaluated tagging different parts of patients' clothes both with respect to the acceptance of healthcare facilities and to the recognition rate of identification and moving direction.

2 System Setup

In order to identify patients and detect their transitions from one room to another we used OBID ID ISC.MR101 mid-range RFID reader [13], multiplexer and two antennas for each door. Antennas are connected to the RFID multiplexer which is connected to the reader that ultimately connects to a PC. Each antenna has a reading range of approximately 30cm and is mounted on the left and right side of a door using free-standing supports that allow changing their height easily. Patients' clothes are tagged also on the left and right side such that moving direction could be recognized (going in or out), deduced by readings on the corresponding antennas (left antenna reads left tag and/or right antenna reads right tag) indicating the direction of passing through the door. In all our experiments (three different locations) door-width was 0.9 – 1m making the reading range of antennas of 30cm suitable fit for the following reasons: a) if the range was considerably larger, the direction of moving is likely to be lost since one antenna might read both tags at the same time, b) if the range was considerably shorter, the antennas might miss both tags. Since the recommended door opening for care facilities may be up to 1.22m [11], the reading range could be adjusted either by using bigger tags (physically larger tags have a greater reading range) or by using the equipment with a slightly bigger reading range.

Clearly, tagging only one side of patients' clothes would be sufficient for detecting the moving direction; however, as expected, the experiments yielded a significant increase in the recognition rate when both sides of clothes were tagged. In the case of a passive RFID system that we used, tags are able to communicate with the reader when in the reading range of antennas and since they do not have a battery, they are smaller in size and less costly than active RFID tags. In the experiments, we used plastic tags with dimensions 8.5x5.5cm affixed on clothes with double sided adhesive tape while for permanent use they might be sewn in the clothes.

3   Evaluation of the Approaches

When it comes to the implementation of RFID-based system for tracking, one must consider various factors that affect the reading accuracy, including tagged objects, tag placement, angle of rotation and reading distance [10]. Moreover, RFID may interfere very often with metal objects in hospital environments. In addition to the technological issues, the key requirement for a system intended for monitoring demented persons is unobtrusiveness, particularly with regards to visible and wearable sensors. Visibility of the RFID equipment is usually a trivial problem (in many cases antennas, readers and multiplexers can easily be hidden from patients) while special attention should be put on tagging strategy since wearable objects may influence patients' activities and they are prone to removing them. However it would be incorrect to consider solely patients as the system's users while not taking into account the healthcare staff. In this respect, choosing the most effective tagging strategy includes identifying the appropriate location for placing tags, their type and size, and a way of attaching tags (permanently or temporarily). The goal is to make an unobtrusive system from the perspective of patients, to minimize the additional workload for healthcare staff and to not interfere with their usual routines while at the same time achieving the highest possible system's accuracy,

The aim of our work was to analyze solutions for tracking demented patients considering the abovementioned constraints and providing an appropriate trade-off between the patient/healthcare staff requirements and the technological limitations. Various possible body locations for placing the tags were examined in accordance with the advices of doctors from a number of rehabilitation centers. According to the caring routines in the centers, doctors' experience with demented persons and the technical constraints, we identified three positions to place passive RFID tags: sole of shoes, hips (pockets of pants) and shoulders of upper garments.

We tested the tracking system in our laboratory, test-bed apartment and a real care facility. The experiments were conducted with two different participants that were passing through the door one after another. The antennas (with a length of 33.7cm) were positioned on the ground, 60cm and 100cm from the ground in the cases of tagging shoes, hips and shoulders respectively. Due to the physical constraints for mounting antennas, the approach of tagging shoes was not tested only in a real care facility. The recognition rates are presented in Fig.1 (minimal and maximal values relate to the highest and lowest system's accuracy concerning different experimental trials). Since it never occurred that a subject was identified while moving direction was missed (and vice versa), the recognition rates are the same for both cases.

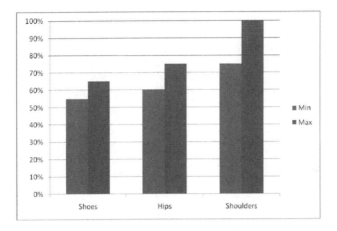

Fig. 1. Moving direction and identification recognition rate

In the case of tagging shoes the system performs at the lowest accuracy mostly due to a higher speed of moving feet than hips and shoulders when a person is walking, providing less time for the RFID reader to identify tags. In addition, in this case the system was more prone to the interference in our experiments, probably because concrete in the floor contained metal objects. On the other hand, tags attached on the shoulders were more parallel to antennas than tags on hips (in most cases in our experiments participants were putting them in their pockets) which resulted in better system's accuracy (putting tags in any other position but parallel with respect to antennas lowers the effective surface for tag-to-antenna coupling).

The type of care facility (daycare or residential nursing homes) can influence the decision of choosing one of the aforementioned places for tagging. In the case of residential care, patients' private clothes can be tagged permanently using waterproof tags (that can be washed with the clothes) sewn in the inner side, in order to be invisible to the patients. Therefore, any of indicated places might suit well so the decision could be based on the criteria of the system's accuracy. Moreover, tagging process may be performed only once which is less time consuming for caregivers. On the other hand, daycare facilities differ more in routines they apply in the sense that some facilities provide clothing (such as shoes or slippers for example) while others allow patients to wear their own. In latter case, it is possible to use tags in form of stickers and attach to patients' clothes upon their arrival. Therefore, in daycare facilities the applied clothing routine should be dominant criteria for choosing an appropriate place for tagging.

4 Conclusion

Tagging shoulders provides the highest recognition rate, being an effective solution for residential nursing homes where it is possible to permanently tag patients' clothes. However, daycare nursing homes differ more in the clothing routines they apply so the tagging strategy depends mostly on this criteria. In these cases, the option is to employ tags in form of stickers that may be attached on hips or shoulders, which provide higher recognition rate for identification and moving direction than tagging the shoes. On the other hand, shoes are often a well-suited place for tagging, since tags remain practically invisible to patients. Therefore, in our future work, we will further investigate the approach of tagging shoes, aiming to increase the recognition rate possibly using different RFID equipment with a higher frequency of reading or multiplexing.

Acknowledgments. The research was funded by the Autonomous Province of Trento, Call for proposal Major Projects 2006 (project ACube).

References

1. Administration of Aging, http://www.aoa.gov (cited December 10, 2010)
2. Dalal, N., Triggs, B.: Histograms of Oriented Gradients for Human Detection. In: International Conference on Computer Vision & Pattern Recognition, vol. 2, pp. 886–893 (2005)
3. Wu, J., Osuuntogun, A., Choudhury, T., Philipose, M., Rehg, J.M.: A Scalable Approach to Activity Recognition based on Object Use. In: IEEE 11th International Conference on Computer Vision, ICCV 2008 (2007)
4. iHygiene Press Release, http://www.woodwardlabs.com/pdfs/iHygiene_Press_Release.pdf (cited December 10, 2010)
5. Ho, L., Moh, M., Walker, Z., Hamada, T., Su, C.-F.: A Prototype on RFID and Sensor Networks for Elder Healthcare: Progress Report. In: SIGCOMM 2005 Workshops (2005)
6. Matic, A., Mehta, P., Rehg, J.M., Osmani, V., Mayora, O.: AID-ME: Automatic Identification of Dressing failures through Monitoring of patients and activity Evaluation. In: 4th International Conference on Pervasive Computing Technologies for Healthcare 2010 (Pervasive Health 2010) (2010)
7. Philipose, M., Fishkin, K., Perkowitz, M., Petterson, D., Fox, D., Kautz, H., Hahnel, D.: Inferring Activities form Interactions with Objects. Context Aware Computing (2004)
8. Kaye, J.: Home based technologies: A new paradigm for conducting dementia prevention trials. In: NIA - Layton Aging & Alzheimer's Disease Center and ORCATECH, the Oregon Center for Aging & Technology. Oregon Health & Science University, Portland (2008)
9. RFID Journal, http://www.rfidjournal.com/article/articleview/4542/1/1 (cited December 14, 2010)
10. Yao, W., Chu, C.-H., Li, Z.: The Use of RFID in Healthcare: Benefits and Barriers. In: IEEE International Conference on RFID-Technology and Applications, RFID-TA (2010)

11. Benbow, W.: Best Practice Design Guidelines for Complex Care Facility (Nursing Home), `http://wabenbow.com/?page_id=16` (cited December 15, 2010)
12. Ashar, B.S., Ferriter, A.: Radiofrequency Identification Technology in Health Care: Benefits and Potential Risks. The Journal of American Medical Association (JAMA) 298, 2305–2307 (2007)
13. FEIG Electronic, `http://www.feig.de/index.php?option=com_content& task=view&id=5&Itemid=59` (cited December 15, 2010)

Processing Location Data for Ambient Intelligence Applications

Samuel del Bello[1], Jared Hawkey[2], Sofia Oliveira[2], Olivier Perriquet[2],
and Nuno Correia[1]

[1] CITI and DI/FCT/UNL, Quinta da Torre, 2829 - 516, Caparica, Portugal
sdelbello@gmail.com, nmc@di.fct.unl.pt
[2] CADA, Ed. Interpress, Rua Luz Soriano, 67, 3°, Sala 43, 1200 - 246, Lisbon, Portugal
jaredhawkey@gmail.com, sofiaoliveira@cada1.net,
olivier@perriquet.net

Abstract. The paper presents contributions in the area of location data processing for pattern discovery. This work forms part of a project which explores an ambient intelligence application designed to present individual users with an overview of their time usage patterns. The application uses location data to build interfaces and visualizations which highlight changes in personal routines, with the aim of stimulating reflection. Data is processed to extract significant places and temporal information about them. The paper presents the questions that can be answered by a data processing layer and the strategy to handle the different types of queries. Location data is processed to identify significant locations, discover patterns and predict future behavior.

Keywords: Ambient Intelligence, Location Data, Clustering, Visualization.

1 Introduction

Mobile devices can capture different types of sensor data, including location and motion, which may be used in context aware applications. Since such devices are carried almost continuously by their users extended data sets maybe readily acquired. The Time Machine project explores personal location data within an artistic context. The goal is to provide each user with an overview of their time usage, identifying routines and extraordinary events. It aims to provide a means for reflection and attempts to present ones habits and personal uses of time. A major component of the project is the construction of mobile interfaces with advanced visualization capabilities. Input data, based on GPS logs, has to be processed to extract relevant and meaningful patterns [1]. This paper focuses on this data processing layer, an essential component for presenting information in meaningful ways. The data processing layer includes a combination of techniques chosen in accordance with the visualization and interface needs, identified as a set of questions the system should be able to answer. A key concern is that the system should run on a mobile device, without resorting to external processing or storage servers, thereby introducing additional constraints on tools used. The paper is organized as follows. The next section presents the

S. Gabrielli, D. Elias, and K. Kahol (Eds.): AMBI-SYS 2011, LNICST 70, pp. 66–69, 2011.

requirements for a data processing layer as a set of questions/queries the system should be able to handle. Section 3 describes the specific technique being implemented, including the identification of significant locations, the discovery of patterns and the prediction of future behavior. The paper ends with conclusions and directions for future work, regarding its integration within a mobile system.

2   Data Processing Requirements

The architecture of the application, developed within the Time Machine project, relies upon a data processing layer that handles location data and provides services to the upper visualization and interaction layers. The requirements for this layer were defined as a set of questions/queries and visualization requirements. This section presents a summary of the processing needs identified. The questions are high level, closer to what a user might request, may contain ambiguities and sometimes need to be decomposed across several data processing functions.

Different time/places/speed usage show different patterns. Here a major concern is to show "different", or extraordinary time usage behavior. The project aims to calculate and represent personal cycles of time, and incorporate what might be considered the natural/human limits of time. Thus, the system will collect data in an ambient manner. The concerns above and the desired functionality to show the routine in terms of the variables being processed: time, speed and places visited, may be further specified and used to provide answers to the following queries, divided in four groups:

1. Is this a new place? Is this a significant place, home/work/other? At which places do I spend more time? Have I travelled a lot today? Which places do I frequent more often?
2. Is this my (usual) pattern for the time of day? Is this my (usual) pattern for this place? Is this sequence of places usual?
3. Is this day different from the norm? Was this a calm/busy day (morning/afternoon)? Was this a long/short day?
4. Where will I go next? Where will I be tomorrow/next week/next month? When will I return to this place?

Each of the above groups will need a different set of tools for location data processing, as described in the next section.

3   Data Processing Tools

This section describes the processing techniques currently being used and the results so far obtained. Some of the questions above, e.g., "Is this a new place?" result from simple data processing, while others like "Is this my (usual) pattern for this place?" require more complex techniques. Preliminary processing aims to find the significant places from the noisy data captured by GPS. Here, raw location data, containing all the data collected by the user, is parsed to extract the approximate semantic notations of location. Fig1 (a), shows such data from a user log as place marks in space.

GPS logs are first parsed into stay points as explained in [3]. This step eliminates non-relevant places and defines those places where the user actually spends time. Fig1(b) shows the stay points parsed from the raw locations. To find the meaningful places for the user, the stay points are clustered using an approximation to the density-based algorithm, DJ-Cluster [4]. Significant places from the previous stay points are shown in Fig1(c). Information about the sequence of places visited is also kept.

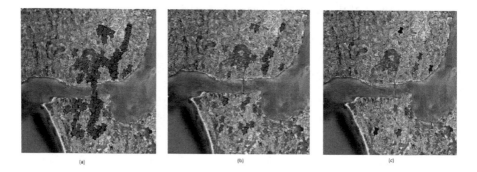

Fig. 1. Two weeks of an user location history: (a) all GPS points from the logs; (b) parsed stay points; (c) meaningful places

Simple statistical data processing using the different dimensions measured provides promising results. The data was processed as described below:

- Daily activity: A time based representation showing whether the individual is moving or stopped. This allows the recognition of daily time patterns, including major changes between states (sleep/awake), and the identification of activity periods.
- Duration and number of visits associated with a location: to identify the most relevant places.
- Features associated with a day: here the idea is to experiment with and study different features of individual days in order to define their signatures, as a first step to cluster and classify days. Currently, the features being tested are the number of visits average/standard deviation, the duration average/standard deviation, stopped time, distance, speed average/standard deviation, and number of visited locations.
- Features associated with an hour: The user behavior can be compared over several days for the same period of the day. The features being tested are distance, speed average, and number of locations visited.

This statistical processing is used to directly support some of the queries mentioned above but also as input for further clustering and classification of the data. Initial approaches to classify and cluster the data have been completed. In concrete, three experiments took place: classify days as weekend/weekday, cluster days and cluster locations. Days were characterized by the durations and frequency of visits to the most relevant locations for that day. These days, labelled as weekends or weekdays were, in some cases, correctly classified in 95% of the cases using cross validation.

The Naïve Bayes classifier was used in this experiment. The X-means algorithm was used for the clustering experiments, due to its efficiency and the advantage of not needing number of clusters as an input; durations and number of visits where also used to characterize the days and the locations. Results show that the days were clustered as expected in many cases but the signature for clusters is still inefficient and further data and tests are required. All experiments were done using the Weka[1] platform.

4   Conclusions and Future Work

The paper presents ongoing work on data processing for a mobile system to show individual time usage patterns. The requirements were identified as a set of queries that the system should answer and current work focuses on testing the processing algorithms. Most of the techniques were identified and tested but further tests with extended sets of data are required. Currently, the project has one dataset for one user with over a year of daily logs, and four shorter data sets each with a few weeks of data. Next, the integration of final versions of the chosen techniques will be developed for the mobile device. With this data processing layer in place, visualizations and interaction options that go beyond the initial proposal [2] will be developed. Regarding additional processing, work is also underway to predict future behavior, using Markov models.

Acknowledgments. We thank DGArtes (The Directorate-General for the Arts of the Portuguese Ministry of Culture) and FCT/MCTES for funding this research as part of the Time Machine project (PTDC/EAT-AVP/105384/2008).

References

1. Ashbrook, D., Starner, T.: Using GPS to learn significant locations and predict movement across multiple users. Personal Ubiquitous Computing 7, 5 (2003)
2. Correia, N., Rodrigues, A., Hawkey, J., Oliveira, S., Amorim, T.: A Mobile System to Visualize Patterns of Everyday Life. In: ISAmI 2011 - International Symposium on Ambient Intelligence, Salamanca, Spain (2011)
3. Li, Q., Zheng, Y., Xie, X., Chen, Y., Liu, W., Ma, W.: Mining User Similarity Based on Location History. In: Proceedings of the 16th ACM SIGSPATIAL International Conference on Advances in Geographic Information Systems, pp. 1–10. ACM, New York (2008)
4. Zhou, C., Frankowski, D., Ludford, P., Shekhar, S., Terveen, L.: Discovering Personal Gazetteers: An Interactive Clustering Approach. In: Proceedings of the 12th ACM SIGSPATIAL International Conference on Advances in Geographic Information Systems. ACM, New York (2004)

---

[1] http://www.cs.waikato.ac.nz/ml/weka

Interactive Haptic Virtual Collaborative Training Simulator to Retain CPR Skills

Prabal Khanal and Kanav Kahol

Department of Biomedical Informatics, Arizona State University
425 N. 5th Street, Phoenix, Arizona, USA
{Prabal.Khanal,Kanav.Kahol}@asu.edu

Abstract. This paper provides a novel approach for training in collaborative environment by integrating collaborative virtual environment (CVE) and haptic joystick. Active World is used as the CVE and Novint Falcon is the preferred haptic device to send force back to the user(s). As our test scenario, we consider cardiopulmonary resuscitation (CPR) skills training simulator for re-training purpose. CPR is not just a compress-and-release procedure - it is a collaborative work and is affected by the performance of each team member. This study also explains the transferability of the CPR skills from this system to the real world case. The data collected from 12 participants verify that this simulator helps users to improve the accuracy of compression rate, and also to retain the skill afterwards.

Keywords: Collaborative Virtual Environment, CVE, Haptics and CVE, Medical education, Collaborative Haptics Training Simulator, CSCW and Haptics.

1 Introduction

Computer Supported Cooperative Work (CSCW) has been a rapidly growing research field after the invention of the Internet. According to Baecker [1], CSCW is an activity, which is performed by groups of collaborating individuals in a computer-assisted environment. He also visualizes CSCW in a form of 2 X 2 matrix of location (local site, different sites) and time (synchronous, asynchronous). Most of the time, CSCW is considered to be a work done by the users located at different sites [2].

Collaborative Virtual Environment (CVE) is generally considered as the combination of CSCW and Virtual Reality (VR) [6]. According to [2], in CVEs, participants share a common virtual environment and are connected to it through a computer network. Participants have their own avatar(s) to represent their identity, location, actions, and gestures. Participants are also able to communicate with each other from within the environment. CVEs are best suited for education as they are capable of providing group discussion (plain text, audio, and/or video), and can also support different media (text, audio, video) to display information about particular topics to the participants. Dickey [5] mentions that a CVE consists of three major components: (a) 3D space illusion; (b) a character to represent real user, called as "avatar"; and (c) an interactive communication environment.

S. Gabrielli, D. Elias, and K. Kahol (Eds.): AMBI-SYS 2011, LNICST 70, pp. 70–77, 2011.

Medical education is, however, slightly different from traditional form of education. Apart from cognitive part of the education, developing psycho-motor skills is also equally important. So far, most of the research on education using CVEs is based on disseminating information to the participants in audio-visual media format. There have been numerous virtual reality based simulators that help the participants learn psycho-motor skills in addition to cognitive skills. However, most of these simulators are standalone and only one participant can access the system. In real world emergency cases, there is a team and each team member has his/her own task to perform. They switch their role back and forth during the same emergency care session. Clearly, this approach of educating medical professionals or medical students is not suited for medical education because not only are the participants communicating with each other, but are also performing psycho-motor activities at the same time.

In this paper, we attempt to solve the issue of collaborative medical education by providing a novel approach of integrating CVE with haptic joystick. This work is a part of advanced cardiac life support (ACLS) procedure, which is a collaborative task, where CPR is one of the most important procedures. In this paper, we focus on the chest compression part of the CPR to re-train the users who have basic idea on how to perform CPR but haven't practiced it for some time. This kind of scenario might occur when clinicians are preparing for continuing medical education although they are not actively performing CPR on patients. Simulators of this kind will be helpful to provide hands on experience in addition to theoretical learning. A participant, who has access to the haptic device, must maintain the rate of 100 compressions per minute while performing CPR on the haptic device. The participant is provided with haptic feedback at real time. Based on his/her performance s/he is given visual feedback in the CVE, so that s/he can improve his/her performance. His/her performance can also be seen by other users who are logged into the system at the same time. This study also intends to check whether the participants retain the CPR skills afterwards.

The paper is organized as follows: we outline related work in Section [2]. The overall system design, methodology, and implementation of the simulator are explained in Section [3]. The experimental design, setup, and participants are described in Section [4]. The results obtain from the simulator are presented in Section [5]. Finally, Section [6] concludes the paper.

2   Related Work

Although CVEs are being used in gaming, socializing, educational as well as working environments [9], only a few selected CVEs can be used in the field of collaborative education. [9], [10] outline different functionalities that should be present in a CVE in order to be suitable for educational purpose.

Boulos, Hetherington, and Wheeler [3] described the potential use of Second Life in medical and health education. They discussed about the use of Healthinfo Island in Second Life for education that is run by a team of information professionals and medical/consumer health librarians. The authors also gave example of virtual neurological education centre (VNEC, www.vnec.co.uk) in Second Life. According to the authors, users were able to learn about neurological disorders by selecting various neurological symptoms in VNEC. The result would be shown by animating their avatars with restriction on their movement and coordination.

Creutzfeldt et. al designed a procedural CPR training system in a virtual world. The authors focused on providing training on various diagnostic steps required during medical emergency. The participants were given questionnaire to get information about the qualitative experience. Based on the response to the questionnaire, the authors mentioned that the training in virtual world offers several advantages.

Pascale, Mulatto, and Prattichizzo [8] proposed and implemented a new idea of using haptic device in a CVE. The idea behind the research was to help blind people to navigate around Second Life with the help of joystick. Instead of visual cues, auditory signals were provided to the users.

To the best of our knowledge, no existing training simulator has been developed for CPR training by integrating haptic device and virtual world, together with the capability of evaluating the performance of the participants.

3 System Design

The design consists of two major components: a CVE, and a haptic device. We used Active Worlds (AW, www.activeworlds.com), which is a CVE and provides its own API that makes it easier for developers to design customized virtual environments. AW allows 30 users to login simultaneously, which provides a platform to perform collaborative work. The haptic device that we used in our system is Novint Falcon haptic device (www.novint.com). The device comes with its own HDAL haptic API that provides different control mechanisms to communicate with the Falcon haptic device. We integrated these two components using their APIs. How the system is developed is explained in sub-section 3.1.

Figure (1) shows the overall design of the system. The direction of the line indicates the information flow.

3.1 Methodology

This research is part of ACLS training simulator in which people work in a collaborative environment. The major objective of this system is to re-train users to perform CPR skills, who already know how to do it, but haven't practiced for some time. Each user's performance is displayed in the CVE (active world). To achieve our goal, we divide the objectives into a set of subtasks.

The first subtask is to calculate force. When participants perform compression, force is calculated and is applied in the opposite direction. The handle of the haptic joystick moves back to the original position, thus simulating 'recoiling'. Mass-spring model is used for its simplicity and efficiency in our system for force calculation. In the proposed system, the force feedback is independent of the visual feedback – it is not necessary to detect collision between the objects in the CVE. This is very important for a collaborative work like CPR because not all members in a team

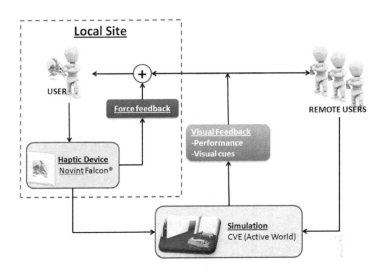

Fig. 1. System Design

perform the same task simultaneously; however, the members switch roles every now and then.

After calculating the force, the number and the rate of compressions are calculated and stored in the local computer, which can be used for the validation of the proposed system.

Once the number and the rate of compressions are calculated, different callback functions, event handlers and attributes provided by Active World SDK are used to visualize the data in the CVE. These data can be seen by all the users who are available at the virtual training location. The output(s) of the system is shown in Figure (2).

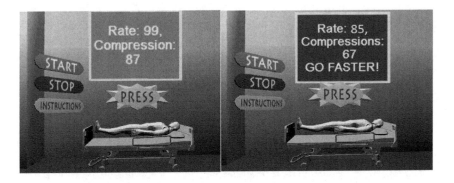

Fig. 2. Screenshots from the system: a) Green board for correct compression-rate, b) Red board for lower compression-rate

4 Experimental Design

Each participant has to perform 3 CPR trials. In the first trial, the participants have to perform CPR without any feedback. They have to maintain the rate of 100 compressions per minute. The second trial provides visual cues and feedback. Participants have to synchronize their rhythm of compression with the visual cues provided on the screen. A 'Press' button is used as a visual cue and it becomes visible and invisible maintaining the rate of 100 per minute. Participants have to perform compression whenever the button appears on the screen, and recoil when it disappears. In addition to the visual instructions, the participants are given feedback on their performance. They are shown their compression-rate, number of compressions and a message (if needed). If their compression-rate is less than 90, then the message "Go Faster!" is displayed, and the participants must increase the rate of compressions. Similarly, when the compression-rate is more than 110 "Go Slower!" message is displayed. These two messages are shown in red background, representing that they are deviant to the actual rate. If their performance is between 97 and 103 compressions per minute, the current compression-rate and the number of compressions are shown on a green background. The third trial is similar to the first one; no visual cues and feedback are provided.

For each trial, the number of compressions, time taken for each compressions (in seconds), and the rate of compression is stored. Our hypothesis is that participants perform better when they are provided feedback (second trial) than when they are not (first trial).

Experiment Setup: 12 participants (3 female, 9 male) participated in the experiment. All participants had basic idea about CPR skills and had already performed CPR before. All of them already knew that they had to maintain the rate of 100 compressions per minute. However, they haven't performed it for 2 months. Only 5 participants had experience on using the haptic device before the study, all others were using the haptic device for the first time.

Before the trials, each participant was explained about the system, the experimental design, and what they had to do in the experiment. Each participant was provided a minute to get used to with the simulator. When they were ready, the first trial was performed. An interval of approximately 0.5 minute separated the trials. Figure (3) shows how the system was set up for the experiment.

5 Results and Discussion

Figure (4) displays the number of compressions in each trial performed by each participant. The safe range (90-100 compressions per minute) is highlighted in the figure. For each trial, performance metrics of each participant, like number of compression, time, and rate of compression, were recorded. Almost 60% of the participants could not maintain their rate within the range of 90-110 compressions per minute. The outcome shows that people who know about CPR, but do not practice it often, tend to make mistake in maintaining the required compression-rate. The

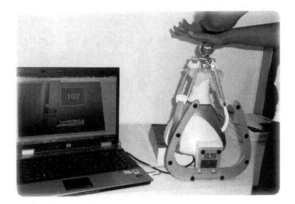

Fig. 3. Experiment Setup: CVE shown at the left and haptic device at the right

compression-rate varied from 76 to 126 per minute.The second trial was performed in presence of visual cues and performance feedback. All participants were able to maintain the compression-rate between 90 and 110. The range of number of compressions per minute varied from 95 to 104 in the second trial. Participants performed better in the third trial as compared to the first one. All of them were able to maintain the compression between 90 and 100. The compression-rate varied from 90 to 110.

We, initially, hypothesized that the participants should maintain the rate between 90 and 110, and providing them the visual cues and feedback would improve their performance. In the visual cues, we displayed their compression-rate, and whether they are going fast or slow, in real time, so that even if they were maintaining the

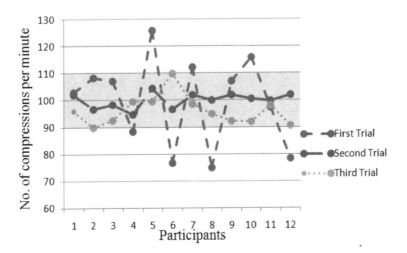

Fig. 4. Performance of 12 participants on each trial (safe-range is highlighted)

required rate, they can improve to maintain it at 100 compressions per minute. Our hypothesis was verified; when they were provided the cues, they performed much better than when they were not given feedback on their performance. The compression-rate varied from 95 to 104, which was more than that we expected.

In the third trial, we wanted to check whether the participants could retain the skill or not if visual cues are not provided. From the outcome of the experiment, we can say that they could retain the skills. All participants could maintain within the range 90-110.

The important thing to mention here is that the participants did not practice on this simulator for a long period of time. Based on the results, even in that short period of time they spent with the simulator, they could retain the skills. It is possible only because they already knew how to perform CPR. This proves that this simulator helps the people, who already know about CPR skills, to perform better by providing feedback on their performance and to retain the skills.

5   Conclusion and Future Work

This paper focused mainly on interactive collaborative CPR skills training simulator for the purpose of re-training the users, who already know how to perform CPR but had not practiced for some time. To achieve our main objective, we also presented a novel approach of integrating haptics and CVE by localizing haptic feedback.

The challenges to design this kind of simulator include the integration of the haptic device to the CVE. As most of the CVEs do not provide application programming interface (API), it is very difficult to integrate with haptics API. Once the haptic device is integrated, it requires very high bandwidth to transmit haptic signals over the internet, which is virtually impossible. This is the main reason to localize haptic feedback.

This opens up different possibilities that we can do with the integration of haptics and CVE. Apart from re-training skilled CPR practitiners, this system can be a part of a virtual mock code training simulator where participants perform different tasks during emergency, and they also need to switch tasks in-between. The participants can log in from different locations, and can interactively practice the mock code in the virtual environment.This can also be used as virtual assessment tool for CPR skills. Participants can log in from a remote site to perform CPR. His/her performance will be stored in a server, where only authorized user can login and evaluate the performance.

The future work includes validation of the learning of CPR skills using the simulator for users who do not have prior CPR experience. As this study was pre-validation of the virtual CPR training simulator, we restricted the number of participants to 12; however, for the validation for unexperienced users, the number of participants will be increased.

References

[1] Baecker, R.M.: Readings in human-computer interaction: toward the year 2000, p. 141. Morgan Kaufmann, San Francisco (1995)
[2] Benford, S., Greenhalgh, C., Rodden, T., Pickock, J.: Collaborative Virtual Environments. Communications of the ACM 44(7), 79–85 (2001)

[3] Boulos, M.N.K., Hetherington, L., Wheeler, S.: Second Life: an overview of the potential of 3-D virtual worlds in medical and health education. Health Information and Libraries Journal 24, 233–245 (2007)

[4] Creutzfeldt, J., Hedman, L., Medin, C., Heinrichs, L., Fellander-Tsai, L.: Exploring Virtual Worlds for Scenario-Based Repeated Team Training of Cardiopulmonary Resuscitation in Medical Students. Journal of Medical Internet Research 12(3), e38 (2010)

[5] Dickey, M.: Brave new (interactive) worlds: A review of the design affordances and constraints of two3D virtual worlds as interactive learning environments. Interactive Learning Environments 13(1), 121–137 (2005)

[6] Kawamoto, A.L.S., Kirner, T.G., Kirner, C.: Experience on the Implementation of a Collaborative Virtual Environment for Educational Applications. In: IEEE International Conference on Systems, Man, and Cybernetics, Taipei, Taiwan, October 8-11 (2006)

[7] Khoury, M., Shirmohammadi, S.: Accessibility and scalability in collaborative eCommerce environments. In: 2nd International Conference on Digital Information Management, ICDIM 2007, vol. 2, pp. 738–743 (2007)

[8] Pascale, M.D., Mulatto, S., Prattichizzo, D.: Bringing Haptics to Second Life. In: Proceedings of the 2008 Ambi-Sys Workshop on Haptic user Interfaces in Ambient Media Systems, vol. (6) (2008)

[9] Tsiatsos, T., Andreas, K., Andreas, P.: Collaborative Educational Virtual Environments Evaluation:The case of Croquet. In: Workshop on Intelligent and Innovative Support for Collaborative Learning Activities

[10] Tsiatsos, T., Konstantinidis, A., Ioannidis, L., Tseloudi, C.: Implementing collaborative e-learning techniques in collaborative virtual environments: The case of second life. In: Fourth Balkan Conference in Title={Implementing Collaborative e-Learning Techniques in Collaborative Virtual Environments: The Case of Second Life, Informatics, BCI 2009, p. 181 (2009)

Future User Centric Media:
Research Challenges and the Road Ahead

Oscar Mayora[*]

NextMEDIA Coordination Action
oscar.mayora@create-net.org
http://www.gatv.ssr.upm.es/nextmedia/

Abstract. This work presents relevant excerpts from two white papers recently published with the support of the Networked Media Unit of the European Commission, outlining a number of research challenges and the way ahead towards providing user centric media, as well as rich multimedia and multimodal content, via the Internet and Ambient Systems over the next decade. It will focus on key advances in Future Media technologies that will enable innovative applications and services, engaging new experiences, where multimedia digital content will be more immersive and closely related to the physical world. According to the consolidated opinion of international experts in the field, high quality research on these challenges will be able to enhance our communication experiences, as well as the way we work and live in the next future.

Keywords: Future Media, User Centric Media, Ambient Media Challenges.

1 Introduction

This work reports relevant excerpts from recent forums and publications supported by the Networked Media Unit of the European Commission, aimed to understand which future challenges need to be addressed by the research and professional community in order to provide user centric media and innovative applications and services through the Internet and Ambient Systems over the next decade.

The first part of the paper will introduce and outline main research challenges in the design of user centric media services in the extended home, where the focus must not be only on the devices and the technologies within the physical home space, but to applications where the user is placed in the centre and allows the home-based services and content to follow the user, regardless of the physical location or the device used for content consumption[1]. It will also address main challenges in the design of personalized access to Media Systems.

The second part of the paper will reflect the consolidated opinion of 25 experts from the EU, USA and Korea consulted by the Future Media Internet Task Force (FMI-TF) on challenges regarding Future Media Technologies, along with the potential impact these challenges might have for the development of Ambient Systems and Media[2].

---

[*] Supported by the Networked Media Unit of the DG Information Society and Media of the European Commission.

[1] ftp://ftp.cordis.europa.eu/pub/fp7/ict/docs/netmedia/user-centric-media_en.pdf

[2] http://www.future-internet.eu/uploads/media/FMI-TF-White_paper_042010_01.pdf

S. Gabrielli, D. Elias, and K. Kahol (Eds.): AMBI-SYS 2011, LNICST 70, pp. 78–106, 2011.

1.1 User Centric Media Services in the Extended Home

The 'connected home' concept has been long researched and solutions that combine communication, audio-visual content and home automation are beginning to appear on the market, promising to simplify the everyday life at home. However, until recently the focus has been on the devices and the technologies within the physical home space. A major breakthrough for user centric media services is taking place nowadays through the delivery and sharing of media content.

Up to now, content was typically broadcasted, to the home, and the users were able to consume it on different home devices, in quite a static manner. The 'extended home' concept places the user in the centre and allows the home-based services and content to follow the user, regardless of the physical location or the device used for content consumption. The user is able to remotely connect to the home and, in a seamless and smooth manner, access the services according to context and profiling. One can consider extending the home network by [1]:

- *Spatial extensions*
  - Users 'taking home with them' when not at home (e.g., access to home information, remote home control)
  - Extending the (closed) home network to multiple homes or home-like sites (office, car, etc.)

- *Functional extensions*
  - Extending the home interface to external services

User centric media services are services created and delivered taking into account the user's preferences and context but also services built by the users themselves.

Such a system is able to assure strong user involvement to co-create their applications by uploading and sharing their user-generated content. The user is not only a content consumer, but also a content creator and distributor.

Sharing of self-created media items can occur among a group of family and friends, or a much wider community/social network.

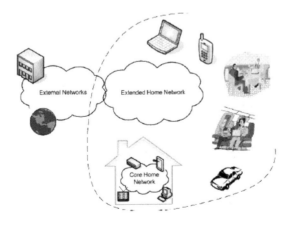

Fig. 1. The Extended Home Concept

1.2 State of the Art

Content distribution channels are changing and the typical broadcast 'one-to-many' model is being redefined.

Large media companies are using alternative methods of distributing their content, including methods that were considered as a threat, in the past. Most music labels sell their content secured with Digital Rights Management (DRM) systems, but some started distributing it also DRM-free, in order to allow users enjoy their legally purchased content on any of their home/mobile devices, without being 'locked' on a specific DRM platform. Traditional TV channels are starting to distribute their programs via Internet peer-to-peer systems.

The Joost service allows users to get a 'TV-like' experience on their personal computers, by leveraging the peer-to-peer distribution, for enjoying content on demand, regardless of their geographical location, or access network. But even the typical television broadcasting experience has become more user-centric by allowing consumers to have control of their preferred time for watching the content. Time-shifting devices and services digitally record programs, from the broadcast television, and have it readily available for users to enjoy at some later point in time, whenever they choose to do so.

Moreover, on-line web-based services, like You-Tube, allow users to easily become active content distributors and reach global audience, by uploading their creations and sharing them with friends or the whole Internet community. Similar initiatives for community oriented content-creation and distribution have been taking place worldwide considering different media channels such as the internet, and most recently through iDTV. Example of this is SAMBA EU project that focuses on generation and distribution of community- oriented content for enhancing inclusion of individuals in society.

As the size of home digital storage devices constantly increases, while their prices keep decreasing, users have the ability to store huge amounts of digital content, both commercial and user-generated, in their homes. Terabyte storage in the home will soon be reality, with such a low cost that no on-line storage service will be able to provide.

In the near future, users will host most of their content in their home network and will access it when away from home, using a mobile device or a remote computer.
The extended home concept, which enables the home content to be accessed from any location depending on the user's preference, is already a reality. Solutions such as the Orb [2] allow the remote access of the home hosted content, from any device that has a web browser. As a PC based solution, it assumes that the home computer is running constantly all day, so that it can serve the remote clients.

At the same time, dedicated stand-alone consumer electronics devices enable the concept of content place-shifting. They are getting the content from the live broadcasted channels, that the user has subscribed to and which are delivered to the home, and encode them to be streamed over the Internet to other personal devices, such as mobile clients. This allows the users to enjoy their favourite television channels, which are available in their homes, as well as in remote locations, in real-time.

Research on personalization, profiling and context awareness has been going on for many years for delivering services and content adapted to the user preferences. [3,4,5]. The mobile world through the 3GPP activities deals with personalization, built on the concept of a Personal Service Environment (PSE), describing how a user can manage and interact with his or her services, and a Virtual Home Environment (VHE), specifying how personalized information can cross network boundaries, thus creating consistency, across multiple devices, with respect to personalized services and features.

In the home environment, there are solutions that allow adaptation of the content to the specific characteristics of the device that will be rendering, mainly focusing on screen size/resolution, supported codecs, etc.

1.3   Gaps and Constraints

Currently, users host their self-generated content in many different locations and devices. Usually, content to be shared with a wider group of friends is uploaded on a 3rd party service, and people are invited to access it from there. More personal content, to be shared only within the family members, is hosted on home devices and there is always content stored on some of the creation devices, like camera phones. For the end users, this fragmentation of content repositories is confusing and difficult to manage.

Hosting content on 3rd party services is efficient, from bandwidth point of view, when the content needs to be shared with a large group of people, but there are always privacy issues.

On the other hand, content that is stored on a home device, which can be accessed via remote access to the home network, is stored on a safe, user-managed, place but, it does not scale for large amounts of visiting users, since remote accessing visitors would cause consumption of the available bandwidth that the home network has. In this way it is clear that there is need for a system that can efficiently and automatically handle the sharing of the user generated content.

Due to the fact that the home network would need to be accessible from the public Internet, for enabling the remote access use-cases, there is a need for a standardized solution. All home devices, regardless of vendor, should be accessible from any kind of personal remote and mobile device.

The access has been given regardless of the Internet Service Provider, that provides the home connectivity to the Internet, or the access network that the remote device uses. Current solutions are proprietary and include many restrictions. Most of them relay either on the fact that homes have publicly accessible Internet Protocol addresses, or that the traffic (between the two end points) is tunnelled via a 3rd party service.

The next generation of the Internet Protocol (IPv6), which has been promising a solution for those two problems for many years, has not been widely deployed yet, and it would bring a new level of administrative complexity in the home, since the direct connectivity to any home device would require much more strict firewall and privacy rules.

The research work that has been done on the personalization area has been focusing on the delivery of the content, which is in the best interest of the user, according to his/her profile. However, the current work on adaptation of the content seems to be focused only on the required transformations to render the media of the preferred device. There is no mechanism to allow, for example, adaptation of the content to fit the time constraints of the user. The reason is that multimedia content is usually treated as a block entity, with just some metadata enhancements. Even worse, if the content is user-generated it is usually lacking metadata, which makes it very difficult to find and adapt after publication.

Recently found European projects are addressing the problems mentioned about in various ways. An example of this can be found in the 6th FP, CONTENT NoE (Content Network and Services for Home Users) whose research goal is to provide seamless, context-aware, end-to-end content delivery in a heterogeneous environment in a community context. This should be possible by addressing the key areas identified as community networks that cover the residential users. A detailed CONTENT research roadmap describes the research challenges in content services, overlay networks and community networks from the point of view of the residential users: CONTENT Deliverable D2.1. 'CONTENT Research Vision and Roadmap' [6].

1.4 Research Challenges

A) Seam less access to content, regardless of its location /repository

User-created content is distributed in many places (online services, home, mobile devices, etc.), and it will always be like this, since every solution has its own advantages and disadvantages, depending on the required usage. One of the key roles that the home intelligence systems could play in the future is the coordination of those resources and repositories. Enabling seamless sharing of all media repositories, between the owner and potential visitors, no matter where the content is really hosted, would be the target. The home, Internet and mobile domain need to merge towards the ultimate user experience, hiding from the users the protocols, interfaces and bearers used for transferring and sharing content. Especially as user generated content size is getting larger in size, due to high resolution cameras, high-definition, etc., the traditional sharing methods (such as MMS, or email) are becoming very limited and unusable.

b) Protecting the digital user experiences, for the future

Clever systems are needed for helping the users automatically backup and archive their content. Nowadays people happily keep a lot of their life-time experiences in digital format, but do not really know how to take care of them, for ensuring that they will not lose them, in case of an accident or a hardware failure.

Unless there is a system in place that can protect the users, and act on their behalf for securing their digital experiences, one will face the sad incidents that people will lose digital experiences (images, videos, etc.) that may have been accumulated over time and the new technology will prove to be much less time resistant than the old traditional methods of storing experiences (e.g. photo paper). Smart homes, mobile devices, storage device and on-line services must form a safety grid for all the user-generated content.

c) How to protect content distribution in the extended home

Digital technology has turned the vision of on-demand content into a reality. With high quality content being so easily transferable, digital content can be enjoyed anytime and anywhere - on any devices of the extended home (TV, DVR, DVD or portable devices).

To ensure that simple and flexible content usage models can be effectively implemented, the industry needs a content protection standard that reflects the needs of all its players:

- *Content providers* want to protect their intellectual property rights against unauthorized redistribution while providing business models that encourage consumption in a secure chain of trust.
- *CA/DRM vendors* want to ensure that the content rights and usage terms defined by their systems are applied to all connected devices in the home network.
- *Device manufacturers and chip vendors* seek an open, low cost solution that promotes device interoperability and a level playing field for competition.
- *Network operators* want to maintain their networks' integrity while ensuring that their consumers can enjoy content on as many connected and unconnected devices as possible.

At the same time, as users start generating more personal content, and share it with their friends, they would like to make sure that it will not leak to others outside their circle of trust. Thus, there is potential need for a DRM system that focuses on user generated content, allowing the creators to set the access and consumption rights for a specific group of people.

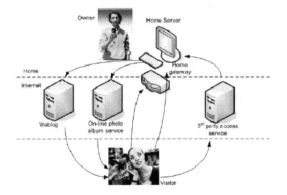

Fig. 2. Current Plethora of Content Offering Methods

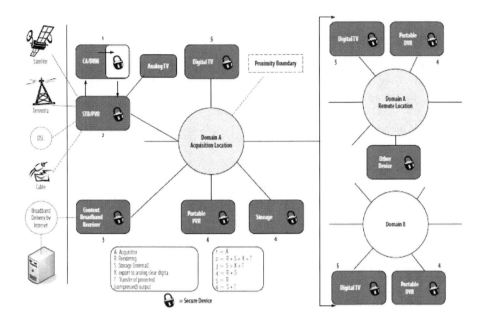

Fig. 3. Secure Domains

d) Content summarization

A new challenge for content adaptation is the method of content summarisation according to the user's profile and time constraints. As users consume content on their mobile devices, away from home, they might have a limited amount of time for viewing some media items. Thus, there is need for intelligent systems that would be able to summarise the content that the user wants to consume, to fit the available time slot that the user has for this. Different media items (e.g. video) can be summarized in order to fit in a smaller time period, without losing essential parts. In such a system, metadata should be inserted through the whole duration of media items, commercial and user created, so that intelligent summarization and optimisation could be carried out based on user mood, available time, and environment context.

e) New user interaction methods in the home

As the activities that the users perform in the digital home are getting complex, there is need for new interaction methods that would allow them to access services and enjoy their content more easily and intuitively. A far more natural interaction between the users and the home devices is required, in order to deliver a personalized experience within the home and the social networks, taking into consideration multiple devices and environments. Research should be focussed on how different kinds of sensors and actuators, such as acceleration, gyroscopes, motion detectors and cognitive cameras, can be used in the home environment for advanced interactive content and context based services. This information, combined with the profiling and context data would allow user interaction via simple, more natural interfaces based on gestures, touch, speech, etc.

1.5 Business Cases / Use Cases

As the home environment becomes more aware about its users and their habits, it will begin making clever decisions on their behalf. Identifying the people that are in the home, their mood and, for example, their next day schedule, the home entertainment system could suggest a list of the most appropriate tv programmes to watch. In the future, users will be able to interact with their media systems, not using a traditional remote control, but maybe just a natural gesture.

These new sets of use cases will require the cooperation and interoperability of multiple in-home and external services. The model of selling stand-alone products and services will be (and is already) transformed to the model of offering experiences, instead.

Users consume content on the mobile devices when they are away from home, for example when commuting to work by public transportation. Depending on the length of their daily trip they might want to watch something on their portable devices, exactly for their duration of their trip, without losing essential information. A clever adaptation system in the home could convert the content in shorter version, to fit exactly the time duration that the user has available.

For example, watching a 45-minute TV series could be cleverly converted into a 35-minute session. Or, watching an originally long personal video clip could become shorter, on demand, by removing parts that are not interesting or are in a way repeated. There is a brand new market of users who are prepared to purchase content if it fits their needs and environment constraints.

New products and services will be offered to the users for automatic management of their content. People will not need to decide anymore what should be stored on the personal computer, what should be backed up on a home storage server, and what needs to be put on on-line services, in order to be shared also with others. The home will be able to support the user by making suggestions and taking some decisions on his behalf, always protecting the content and the privacy of the creators.

Automated backup and archiving will ensure that data is always replicated on a secure location, while clever synchronization mechanisms will make sure that the latest content will be available to the users when using their mobile/portable devices when outside the home. Also, remotely connecting to the home network will become an intuitive and transparent task for users that will not notice explicit differences when accessing data regardless where the content that they consume is located. New market space is created for service providers that will be handling the management and security complexity of the home networks, on behalf of the users.

1.6 Potential Research Themes

The areas which are of particular interest, in the extended home domain, could be some of the following:

- Seamless content access and sharing, regardless of the location of the content (home or externally hosted).

- Mash-up of home and external service. The home providing web-service interfaces to other Internet services, for ultimately personalized experiences.
- The home as the last place of privacy. How to keep it this way?
- Systems for automated backup and content loss prevention.
- New user interaction methods, in the home environment.
- Ambient telepresence and hybrid physical/digital presence.

1.7   Personalised Access to Media Systems

As the available amount of data is constantly increasing, the need for finding accurate and relevant information quickly becomes a necessity. Given that knowledge worker spend a large amount of time in searching for the right information, any mechanism to reduce this time spent will have a large impact. This aim has lead to a growing interest in personalization techniques.

Personalization is the use of technology and user information to tailor interactions between a service or task and each individual user according to the user's perceived or stated preferences. Using information either previously obtained (e.g. interests, occupation, hobbies, etc) or provided in real time about the user (relevance feedback), the offerings of the system are altered to fit the user's stated or inferred needs.

Personalized access is generally described as the system's ability to customize the user interface, the information channels and the services provided according to the individual user's needs, personal interests and preferences.

Personalization is one of the key elements towards achieving success of user centric media services, both in terms of producing and sharing (and/or searching and retrieving) content. The vision is to create a user centric media landscape, in which user creativity and user experience is placed on the forefront.

User creativity is encouraged, and user created content reaches its envisaged audience, by means of developing new ways to find, access and consume ready-made or individually tailored media. New forms of entrepreneurship might arise and existing enterprises will be able to refine their offering enhancing their business or making them more competent by focusing on specific niches.

1.8   State of the Art

The average European user is already in possession of several intelligent devices; this can be seen as an essential shift in modern European lifestyle. It is important to remember that the success of these technologies is strongly related to sociological factors. For each device, a user usually receives and uses content tailored to the specific device.

We come to a point where one can assume that personalization can be categorized into aspects of personalized service and personalized interface. Personalization till now has mostly been perceived as a way to change the look or behaviour of the device (personalized interface), for example ring tones or themes for mobile phones or customisation of popular video and audio players.

However, a personalized service environment would present the key for mass adoption of networked media services, as it would offer users very strong 'socializing' tools. User-produced content would reach its audience easier and User Centric Media approaches would bridge the gap between available technology and 'social' needs.

Several Technologies and approaches, which are already available today, have to be considered when it comes to developing new aspects and trends of User Centric Personalization.

These include aspects of the user device, aspects of the user preferences, requirements (content and context), privacy and aspects of media management (device and content).

Semantics and context also play a critical role in personalization. In today's increasingly dynamic media environments, adequate information about media files and their domain relations and services is essential to allow for user centric media to be accessible and to maintain a certain degree of navigation between the huge amounts of available material.

Ongoing research in technologies related to user, context and device profiling have already resulted in some degree of commercially mature products, for example user profiling in several sites, is using data collected from a number of different sites, which can result in the creation of a personalized web page. Service, content and device providers can leverage this user-specific knowledge to offer products that allow individualized and navigable content query and retrieval. Technologies used include content-based and collaborative filtering, in which a filter is applied to information from different data sources to select relevant data that may apply to the specific (usually e-commerce) experience of a customer or specific group of customers.

The difference between the two lies in the process of identifying the content that is suitable for the user. When using content-based filtering, the suitability of a particular content for a user is estimated through direct comparison of content meta-data and the model of the active user. When using collaborative filtering, the similarity between users is estimated first, and content that is liked by users similar to the active user, is recommended. Both approaches can be used as complementary methods, as both have advantages and drawbacks. Finally, data analysis tools are also used to predict likely future interactions.

User Profiling has also become the prime task of specific consulting companies that collect information about user habits to allow content providers to better target their audiences.

Since personalization depends on gathering and using personal information about the user, adequate protection of users' privacy is a major concern.

1.9 Gaps and Constraints

Currently, personalization is exploited mostly by businesses in order to allow for making consumer-provider relationships more closely tailored to the individual. The perception is solely driven by means of marketing and sales. The user is perceived simply as a consumer, and a sound personalization strategy exists only to improve customer service.

Although profitable businesses have the means to enrich their customer base by using existing technologies, user centric media approaches have different needs and different goals. It's not sufficient to personalize the end-user and remember their name, but to place context in the equation and to ensure both creative and interface are appropriate for the individual. Personalization then would allow tailoring the level of richness and productivity to create a well-rounded approach for users to interact with each other and also for businesses to interact with the users.

Another important issue is the search and retrieval of the requested material. Users get annoyed by situations that limit their control on the content they receive. The user will, for example, not be satisfied with a slow service response due to networks with low transmission rate, or a service presentation layout that does not fit the display of the user terminal, or get thousands of document titles as a result of an information search. From the service provider's side it is not possible and economical to make different versions of a service for every different terminal type and network.

Unlike conventional text-based search, media (audiovisual) search tasks usually aim at retrieving something similar to a query. In addition, the query specification and resources to be searched are often of different media types, e.g., the query is formulated in terms of keywords (text) and the retrieved resources are images, sound, video, etc. On the other hand, the query itself may be complex consisting of multi-components of different media types. As a consequence, it is usually difficult the express the query precisely. There are often ambiguous mappings between query description and its underlying interpretation.

To capture the user's real intention of audiovisual search, the query usually needs to be properly interpreted in an interactive way. It is more often a result of several iterations of interpretation and refinement.

Recommender Systems were originally defined as systems in which 'people provide recommendations as input, which the system then aggregates and directs to appropriate recipients'. Current generation of recommender systems still requires further improvements to make recommendation methods more effective and applicable to an even broader range of real-life applications, including recommending multimedia content or products to purchase in a store made by a 'smart' shopping cart.

These improvements include better methods for representing user behaviour and the information about the items to be recommended, more advanced recommendation modelling methods, incorporation of various contextual information into the recommendation process, utilization of multi-criteria ratings, development of less intrusive and more flexible recommendation methods that also rely on the measures that more effectively determine performance of recommender systems. Furthermore, most algorithms focus on single item recommendations and do not consider any more complex recommendation structures.

Finally, since personalization depends on personal information about the user, which must be collected and stored by the system, there is a major issue regarding adequate protection of the user's privacy. Up to now, the real identity of the user is mostly concealed behind a pseudonym, which is associated with all user-related information stored by the system.

This implies that the user has somehow registered with the system and must log on to it in order to access his personalized interface. Even though no real identity can be connected with the pseudonym, this doesn't prevent misuse of user information in all cases. An example is targeted advertising, which does not need to know who the user really is, but is only interested in knowing that the user that is now logged on is known and has a specific profile.

1.10 Research Challenges

a) Adaptive Multimedia Content and Dynamic Personalized Composition of Multimedia Content

Content Adaptation up to now refers to the action of transforming content to adapt to device capabilities.

Content adaptation is usually related to mobile devices that require special handling because of their limited computational power, small screen size and constrained keyboard functionality.

However, effective personalization schemes have to be researched in order to lead to the creation of adaptive content not only in terms of content format but also in terms of content context. Research Items include:

- Semantic-based, personalized delivery concept.
- Adaptation of content based on user experience and perceptional factors. Adaptation of either content or service to achieve the perceptional quality of experience required by each individual user.
- Shifting of multimedia adaptation functionality to Web Services accessible through standard interfaces that allow for multimedia format conversion and composition leading to flexible, application independent adaptation.
- Agent technologies for automated Web service discovery, execution, composition, and interoperation. They present a logic-based agent technology for service composition, predicated on the use of reusable, task-specific, high-level generic procedures and user-specific customizing constraints.

Future research should also aim at the development of technologies and tools to continuously monitor and improve the overall quality of media services.

The outcome of this research (technology and tools) is intended to be implemented in both popular, commercial (e.g. triple-play market, mobile services) and specialized (e.g. medical digital video libraries) services.

The most innovative and prominent functionality is expected to be the introduction feedback mechanisms allowing not only for Quality of Experience (QoE) assessment and monitoring but also for QoE improvement (long-term QoE improvement with network infrastructure and QoS parameters modifications and short-term QoE improvement with flexible content compression, transcoding and adaptation).

In terms of content adaptation, expected diversity of end user content reception devices should also facilitate introduction of content adaptation services, such as compression schemes with new generation time-varying Compression Ratios (CR). Varying in time compression ratio can be applied to a recording in which some parts are of higher importance than others.

b) Efficient Content Search and Retrieval

User centric personalized access to media systems should allow for a very efficient way of locating the desired information based on user preferences and user profiles.

Given the option to fine tune search and retrieval preferences, user centric media approaches will ease the way of locating and retrieving information in environments characterized by immensely large amounts of data and content, either professional or user created and available in single or distributed environments.

Today, even the most advanced methods of content retrieval cannot prevent avalanches of query results coming down to the user, whereas the user would like only the most 'relevant' content displayed. In order to overcome these issues, the following technologies should be further researched:

Methods for modeling users
User interaction mechanisms should provide observation mechanisms, based on which conclusions can be obtained about user preferences. Related to these mechanisms is the type of user relevance feedback that is obtained. Users should be able to evaluate the suitability of a particular content or the system may have to make implicit assumptions based on user actions on the content.

Semantic-based content search with support for content distribution networks
P2P computing is a potentially powerful model for information sharing between ad-hoc groups of users because of its low cost of entry and natural model for resource scaling. As P2P communities grow, however, locating information distributed across the large number of peers becomes problematic. Further research is required in adapting state-of-the-art algorithms, to content sharing environments and to the formulation of multiple communities with cross-interests.

Content-based search is expected to become the next big trend in search engines. These technologies allow the indexing (annotation) and querying of real visual (image, 3D) or acoustic information inside multimedia content and are based on very advanced recognition and segmentation algorithms.

User Centric Media systems will especially benefit from this technology, since it would allow classification of content that is lagging completely metadata annotations or is incorrectly tagged (sometimes on purpose).

Combinations of semantic and content-based search
The introduction of automatic tagging procedures based on low level optic/acoustic characteristics of media files. The latter assumes specific research on the combination of low-level characteristics, which constitute the basis of content-based retrieval, with high-level semantic interpretations of the content in a structured manner (using for example specific ontologies).

Most of the aforementioned research topics concerning content/context based search and retrieval of 3D content are covered by the project VICTORY (www.victory-eu.org), while project DIVAS (www.ist-divas.eu) is effectively researching indexing and direct search techniques for compressed audio and video files.

c) User Privacy

Future systems should address *User Privacy* issues carefully than currently considered. User information should be treated according to easily understandable policies that users have easy access to. Trust mechanisms should exist, that allow users to verify that systems use their information according to the agreement.

Users should be able to look into the data that has been collected about them, modify it, remove it, and even personalize the data collection policies themselves. Development of standards in this direction would help greatly, as they intend to ensure interoperability between devices and trust by the users.

Convenience and security are always competing aspects of systems of any kind. There is a great challenge in designing systems that are both secure and easy to use. Novel user centric media systems should be both.

d) Content Mobility, Accessibility and Convergence of Networks

Today, mobility is of significant importance. With the introduction of wireless networks the user has become increasingly mobile, freeing himself from the bounds of a fixed connection to the internet, and thus, to the system. Therefore, content produced by the user becomes mobile as well, a fact that raises issues when needing to keep it always accessible to other users of the system.

Content Mobility and Accessibility is therefore a research challenge on its own, in three main areas:

- Provision of tools, services and systems for supporting mobile user creativity and content production (produce and share on the move).
- Efficient content adaptation, transmission, storage and sharing for addressing the largest possible audience.
- Value added services of a converged media and networks. This is a challenge for content distribution networks, especially for personalized access to content, because the ways into which content can be acquired and used are multiplied by this convergence.

e) Content protection

Copyright protection (or Ownership appreciation) of the content and insurance of the content ownership are of significant importance in creating user-centric repositories. So far two main complementary research areas seem to provide the necessary protection both for the content and for the owner: watermarking and Digital Rights Management (DRM). Watermarking techniques have long been used for the provision of robust copyright protection of multimedia material as well as for multimedia annotation, with indexing and labeling information.

The main challenge in content watermarking is the robustness of the watermarking techniques against several types of attacks that do not substantially degrade the model's visual quality such as rotation, translation and uniform scaling, points reordering, remeshing, polygon simplification, mesh smoothing operations, cropping, local deformations.

DRM allows intellectual property owners to express policies for content usage with confidence that these policies will be respected once the content is distributed in the network. Integration of P2P technology with DRM is the latest and possibly the most important technological and business frontier and it is partly faced in the project VICTORY.

1.11 Business Cases/Use Cases

As the users become the centre of interest and gain more power, both user communities and business communities gain from this experience. Combining the best of both worlds', users will finally be able to personalize their 'experience'. From interface and device to content a new media production and consumption environment arises, that serves technological and social advancement alike.

Tailored multimedia content is delivered seamlessly to multiple devices. Users will be able to indicate a preference for a particular content type or types, and content will be chosen or even created, based on user preferences.

Users may further refine content preferences as content is experienced, thus having a more enjoyable experience.

Search results, based on content and semantic characteristics, will be more efficient and more productive. In commercial scenarios users will be able to find and indicate a desire to purchase content or learn more about specific content. Searching through a vast amount of information will become easier and huge niche markets will evolve in which all content can reach its intended audience.

User feedback on the 'Experience' will be considered to enhance future services, from content production to sharing and consumption.

2 3D Content Generation Leveraging Emerging Acquisition Channels

Content creators always look for new forms and ways for improving their content and adding new sensations to the viewer experience. High Definition video has been the latest innovation in the area of content enrichment. 3D is the next single greatest innovation in film-making. Recent film releases such as 'Avatar' have revolutionalised cinema by the extensive use of 3D technology and 3D content production along with real actors creating a new genre at the outset of the 2010s. The box office tickets show that audiences have very quickly embraced this by making Avatar the most successful in cinema ticket sales film in the history of digital cinema (beating even the Titanic).

However, today's young society is becoming increasingly content art and design "literate" as a result of technological advances and lower costs in photography, cinematography, 2D/3D graphics design and animation technologies and as a result of increased emphasis on media design in education. As a result, novel forms of 3D content, should also find its way into small and medium size content creation companies, moving the experience from cinema halls and cinema projectors to the everyday household environments and computers, providing increased number of audiences with a taste of the versatility and power of 3D as both consumers and producers. 3D Internet is a concept that has recently come into the spotlight in the R&D arena, catching the attention of many people, and leading to a lot of discussions. Several research challenges such as: visualisation and representation of information, and creation and transportation of information, among others, will need to be investigated and solution found for 3D internet to become a reality.

The success of 3D cinema has led to several major consumer electronics manufacturers and broadcasters to announce plans to launch 3D-capable TVs and offer 3D content in 2010. 3DTV will require the integration of a diversity of key technologies from computing to graphics, imaging to display, and signal processing to communications.

There are a number of competing 3D technologies available, and the decision to support 3D will require an understanding of the relative merits of each in the context of the home. The provision of 3D content into the home will require significant cooperation between content providers, service providers and consumer electronics manufacturers to ensure consumer confidence in the technology and avoid a repeat of the confusion surrounding the introduction of HD technologies.

Today's 3DTV technology is based on stereo vision where left and right eye images are presented to the viewer through temporal or spatial multiplexing by wearing a pair of glasses. Usually the content is captured using two cameras mounted on a rig. Recently there are few consumer electronics manufacturers that provide a single camera set up for the capture of the left and right eye images. The next step in the 3D TV development could be the multiview autostereoscopic imaging system, where a large number of pairs of video signals are recorded and presented on a display that does not require glasses for viewing. Although, several autostereoscopic displays have been reported, there are still limitations on resolution and viewing position. Furthermore, stereo and multiview technologies rely upon the brain to fuse the two disparate images to create the 3D sensation. As a result such systems tend to cause eye strain, fatigue and headaches after prolonged viewing as users are required to focus to the screen plane but converge their eyes to a point in space, producing unnatural viewing.

With recent advances in digital technology, some human factors which result in eye fatigue have been eliminated. However, some intrinsic eye fatigue factors will always exist in stereoscopic 3D technology.

Creating a truly realistic 3D real-time viewing experience in an ergonomic and cost effective manner is a fundamental engineering challenge. Future 3D technology should seek to advance the current existing technologies not only in capturing and manipulating 3D content but also in creating a new 3D content format which offers fatigue free viewing with more than one person independently of the viewer's position.

3D holoscopic and holography are two technologies that overcome the shortcomings of stereoscopic imaging, but their adoptions for 3D TV and 3D cinema are still in their infancy. Holographic recording requires coherent light but offer the ultimate 3D viewing experience. Holoscopic video uses microlens arrays to recording a 3D scene and can operate under incoherent illumination, which is in contrast with holography, and hence it allows more conventional live capture and display procedures to be adopted.

Future 3D video could use different technologies for 3D content creation and display.

2.1 Future Research Challenges

Communicating information using images plays a major role in today's society. There are a significant number of applications where the ability to display and visualize a

3D image comfortably confers real benefits. Examples from the professional domain include medical imaging, scientific visualization, security/defense, education, computer-aided design, and remote inspection. While in consumer markets 3D video games and 3D multimedia offer a rich experience to the consumer.

In very recent years 3D technology has become an extremely hot topic of research and there is a real feeling of excitement surrounding the technology. With the success of 3D movies such as Avatar burned in their memories, content creators, distributors, consumer electronics manufacturers and Hollywood studios have all expressed serious interest in wowing their own audiences. As a result, research in the 3D technology has intensified to progress its introduction to the home consumer be it 3D TV and/or 3D internet. However, for the 3D technology to be fully adopted by the home consumer, solution to several research challenges need to be investigated and solutions are needed to simplify the generation of 3D content and provide the users/ producers similar hardware and software facilities as those enjoyed today by 2D video makers and users. Among other research challenges, visualization and representation of information, and transportation of information, remain key despite the numerous advances made in the field of stereo vision.

3D content generation

Today, the capture of 3D images and video relies on stereo vision where a number of cameras located in different positions are used. However, this kind of setup for 3D content production is cumbersome and requires correct calibration of all cameras. To that effect an important research challenge is to develop novel technologies which allow the 3D content to be captured using a single 3D camera and hence simplifies 3D video production and allows adoption of the well known techniques used today in 2D video production.

Due the increasing in computing power, computer generated graphics are becoming more and more an essential part of today visual content. Hence another research challenge is provide repositories of reusable and adaptable 3D assets (animated characters, background/environments, props, etc) that can communicate/ interact with each other and systems that share/distribute rendering and processing requirements over intelligent networks. Computer graphics plug-ins have been developed for the generation of stereo images. However, if a new 3D content genre is defined to avoid the shortcomings of stereo imaging, then similarly true 3D graphic tools need to be made available.

3D Content Editing, Authoring and Sharing

The dramatic explosion of the user-generated content culture on the web has illustrated that any new form of 3D content should be able to take off on non professionals online resources such as YouTube. This would allow both professional and non-professional authors to jointly develop 3D content with a more realistic sensation. Tools are required for users, whether professionals or not, to be able, via open source authoring environments, to create intelligent content but also to share it across open networks and remix it by using various elements of different distributed content items to produce in turn new content.

There exist a wealth of software tools available today to home consumer for editing and authoring of 2D audio visual content. Hence, it is a requirement that similar tools are made available to the home consumer as well as professionals to allow editing and authoring for seamless compositing of any new form of 3D content. The interconnecting backbone of today's World Wide Web is still the hypertext. Although a plethora of multimedia content is published on the internet, non-hypertext interactivity is sandboxed on the site. In order to create a real 3D Internet experience, hyperlinks must not be restricted to the hypertext, but extended to any kind of media available on the internet (hypermedia). In 3D video, extraction of objects is potentially easier, as parallax effects clearly separate foreground objects from the background. These objects can be used to link to further 3D video clips, allowing for nonlinear video experiences.

3D Visualisation

Binocular vision feed the human brain at all time with slightly offset views of a scene: the greater the disparity, the closer the object. At the same time, converging nearby or far away gives our brain hints of distances. This principle has been exploited by stereo vision technique where two discrete views are presented to the left and right eye of the viewer via colour, polarisation or time separation techniques requiring special glasses. Over the last few years a number of autostereoscopic multiview 3D displays have been demonstrated where lenticular optical elements or parallax barriers technologies are used to separated the left and right view.

A particularly contentious aspect of stereoscopic displays for entertainment applications is the human factors issue. Furthermore, due to the lack of perspective continuity in 2D view systems, objects in the scene often lack solidity (cardboarding) and give rise to an 'unreal' experience. Hence for 3D TV and 3D internet to become a reality, another research challenge that needs investigating and resolving is the development of 3D content format and related technologies which offers fatigue free viewing with more than one person independently of the viewer's position.

3 Immersive Multimedia Experiences

Traditionally, research on multimedia has provided information to the user primarily through just two sensory modalities - sound and vision. Hence up to now, research on different aspects involving multimedia from coding, to transmission to evaluation of the quality of experience and interaction has mainly been focused on these topics. Although there is a growing interest in other types of sensory interaction such as haptics, sound and in general more immersive experiences of multimedia, the topic is still under researched. This statement is even more valid for research on aspects related to the integration, display and transmission of multisensory information enriching the multimedia experience.

Research on immersive multi-sensory environments has proven that taking into account multisensory data such as vibro-sensory (e.g. floor vibration) and low-frequency subsonic effects could improve distance communication in applications like remote music performance and telemedicine. However, still no advanced strategies for data compression and transmission of these alternatives modalities have been adopted.

Other research is focusing on alternative and novel ways for interacting with media, e.g. through tangible interactions and use of natural elements.

Regarding the development of new user interfaces, recent research on immersive displays has made relevant progress related to instruments for surround-view and high definition cinema for designing more engaging immersive experiences. Other approaches of immersion consider a shift from highly structured settings of interfaces (like virtual reality and large screens) to more portable ones such as mobile devices augmenting the real world. An important research aspect in all these new interactive systems is pushing interaction designers to exploit the intrinsic characteristics of immersiveness to improve intuitiveness in interaction to enhance user experiences.

Nowadays, the research on immersive interactions has provided a series of applications at the level of the state-of-the-art with high potential of providing social benefit to users and better life quality. Examples of these are in the field of therapeutic systems and rehabilitation, exertion games, connectedness, locative media for education and digital TV among others. To not underestimate is the important issue that is rising among social scientist regarding immersive environments is the perception and relevance of aesthetics in such environments or more critical, the social implications of these new applications amongst which potential addictions to technology-based experiences.

Other relevant work relies on the concept of Social Immersive Media. The notion of this concept has been formalized recently5 in the context of multimedia immersive museum exhibits, by extrapolating a trend enabled by advances in the technology of interacting games, direct manipulation interfaces, and interactive arts.

3.1 Future Research Challenges

We live in a multimedia world. Users are increasingly looking for new multimedia experiences: new ways to capture, share and consume their multimedia content. In recent times, both research and industry has focused on designing technology that could enable immersive experiences with multimedia content, especially suited for home environments. These environments might enable the users to interact with multimedia content even when they are not co-located.

Despite many years of research on Media Spaces, we are still far from developing technologies that would allow people to virtually interact at distance with the same efficiency and ease than when face-to-face. Ethnographical observations from real work settings show that many solutions developed to support collaborative interactions at a distance are flawed as they "fracture the relation between action and the relevant environment". For example, using many video cameras to capture and share different points of view between two remote locations might seem to be an improvement over the use of a single camera. However, users might feel lost in the attempt to understand which view is the partner currently looking at or how to adapt common communication strategies to this multitude of perspectives. We need to find more subtle technological solutions to translate communication mechanisms which are effective in presence but not available when conversational partners are not co-located. These solutions should allow recreating the same functions using different but equivalent strategies. We highlight a number of these mechanisms that might potentially enable unexplored interaction capabilities in media spaces.

Gesture recognition

It is well known that gestures complement verbal interactions and help humans to disambiguate references used during the interaction (e.g., discussing blood test reports from different patients) or to better support comparisons between various information media (e.g., combining a broken leg x-ray result with a plastic leg miniature so that the physician can point specific articulations in the former and manipulate the latter while explaining the injury cause). Supporting and developing new approaches to gesture recognition is of primary importance for immersive multimedia experiences.

Advanced Gesture recognition also helps in enhancing the user QoE.

Modeling the focus of attention

One of the challenges that designers of interactive immersive environments are constantly facing is the detection of the users' focus of attention. This roughly corresponds to the point in the shared workspace that is currently looked at by the user and/or the objects s/he is interacting with.

Detecting this element is extremely complicated. However, this information is extremely valuable as it can help designers design better support systems for the users' interactions in the system. Future immersive multimedia spaces will benefit from sensors and models able to recognize the users' focus of attention. In this context, the eye contact could be advantageous, where most of the existing means for remote interaction (e.g., video conferencing, web cams, etc.) do not allow the eye contact, where each user should focus on the camera, which does resemble the nature communication.

Context detection and modeling

Future Internet Media devices should react in a dynamic fashion to changes in the user's situation, for instance switch automatically from visually displaying text to reading the text out loud when the user starts another activity that keeps him/her from looking, yet not from listening. Time-saving applications would be very helpful as well. Any modality of content (including 3D, haptic content, games, etc.) and its delivery should be intelligently substitutable at any time, for reasons of convenience, time-saving, filtering for relevance, or improved understanding - not to mention bandwidth bottlenecks or the benefits of people with disabilities.

3D body reconstruction

Advancements in the field of video analysis might allow in the near future to design immersive environments where the 3D model of the body of the user is fully reconstructed from the video feed of several cameras available in the environment. From this information more elaborated task models can be derived and used to allow forms of interactions with computational devices and multimedia content. With the development of 3D human body scanners, it becomes possible to generate hundreds of accurate body measurements as well as an accurate 3D shape (without skeletal knowledge) in the form of point clouds from a specific subject. From this information a complete pipeline will allow capturing the shape of real people with parameterization techniques for modeling to animation. Furthermore, comprehensive biomechanical models can offer accurate mechanical body deformability through an accurate, however complex representation of the biologic materials below the skin (muscles, fat tissues, bones) and how these interact between each other.

Integration of digital and physical space

In media spaces, humans tend to interact with both digital and physical artifacts. However, connections between these two realms have been limited so far. One of the challenges for the future of these environments will be to build better support and easy translation between "bits and atoms".

Furthermore, the goal would be to not only recreate and emulate face-to-face setting but to design interaction capabilities that can be augmented by technology enabling forms of interactions that are not possible in standard co-located interactions.

Persuasive multimedia experiences

Immersive multimedia environments might not only provide new ways of creating and consuming media for entertainment or work purposes. Combined with persuasive technologies, these environments might stimulate users towards a positive change in their behavior (e.g., embracing a more active lifestyle, etc.).

Multisensory immersive experiences

Today immersive systems are mostly focused on audio-visual applications while other sensorial modalities are still largely uncovered. While for audio and video there exist extensive studies employing models of human perception (e.g. for advanced compression, interaction, etc.), multisensory data is only marginally considered.

Social Immersive Multimedia (SIM)

SIM is a form of computer generated/mediated augmented reality that focuses on the aspects of social (interpersonal) interactions and aims at overcoming the still dominant GUI (Graphic User Interface) metaphor in multimedia. SIM aims at providing immersive experiences (including for example: communication, education, entertaining, training, and socialization) to users by means of body controlled interactivity, using lightweight (even invisible) sensing infrastructures, rather than cumbersome wearable technologies.

Ultimately the goal is to design user interactive behavior so to attain highly effective and engaging experiences at a social level. SIM is an emerging research area in the Human Computer Interaction (HCI) research community whose value and impact (economic and social) will be boosted by its incorporation in the framework of the Future Internet Multimedia. In particular the open, scalable, ubiquitous Future Media Internet infrastructure coupled with Social Immersive Multimedia will open the way to the formation of a new generation of Internet based services for consumers and of user-centric social networks.

4 Multimedia, Multimodal and Deformable Object Search

Multimedia content, which is available over the Internet, is increasing at a rate faster than the respective increase of computational power and storage capabilities. Internet capacity will approach the amount of yota (1024) bytes in 2010. Such a tremendous amount of content cannot be processed and indexed by the current computational power unless personalised and user-centric mechanisms are implemented so that only the content of interest is delivered to the end-users.

This growth of popularity of media is not accompanied by the rapid development of media search technologies and the existing solutions still lack several important features, which could guarantee high-quality search services and improved end-user experience. These features are listed below:

Multimodal content search and retrieval in a unified manner

Currently, information is perceived, stored and processed in various forms leading to vast amounts of heterogeneous multimodal data (ranging from pure audiovisual data, to fully enriched media information associating also data originating from real world sensors monitoring the environment, etc.). User perception and interpretation of the information is in most cases on a conceptual level, independently of the form this content is available. Assuming the availability of an optimal, user-centric, search and retrieval engine, when users search for content they should be able to:

- express their query in any form most suitable for them;
- retrieve content in various forms providing the user with a complete view of the retrieved information;
- interact with the content using the most suitable modality for the particular user and under the specific context each time.

Sophisticated mechanisms for interaction with content

Secondly, social and collaborative behaviour of users interacting with the content should be exploited at best, which will enable them to better express what they want to retrieve. We need to pay a great research attention on increasing the content utilization efficiency, measured as the fraction of the relevant delivered content (i.e., content which satisfies their information needs and preferences) over the total amount of delivered content.

Towards the direction of delivering relevant multimedia content to users, another barrier that needs to be overcome is that the vast amount of information is not actually annotated.

Efficient presentation of the retrieved results

Search results suffer in most cases from the sequential presentation and the information overload, i.e. the presentation of huge amounts of information which is in most cases irrelevant to the query or not optimally presented to the user. This becomes significantly more important when information search and retrieval is performed from mobile or notebook devices with limited presentation capabilities. Appropriate filtering of the retrieved results is needed combined also with advanced visualisation techniques to compress information utilising the visual space and novel interfaces for fast and easy information access, based on context aware information, such as location and device specific performance indicators.

Efficient methods for deformable objects search and retrieval

In most of the multimedia object retrieval approaches presented so far, search is performed by using as query a similar object. Low-level feature extraction methods are applied to the object, providing a description of the object's global shape. These methods are not sufficient for Future Media Internet applications for three main reasons:

- An input multimedia object is not always available and it cannot be created from scratch by a non-expert user. On the other hand, using as query an image/video or a hand-drawn sketch is more convenient (e.g. a 2D photo can be taken from the mobile device's digital camera; a sketch can be drawn by using a PDA touch screen interface, a low-quality audio excerpt can be recorded from the mobile phone, etc.).
- Neither partial matching nor articulation invariance is supported by methods applied to the (3D) objects' global shape. Articulation invariance is essential for applications where deformable objects exist (usually fashion applications).
- Presently introduced multimedia search engines commonly do not allow the user to form complex and multi-modal queries. While the multimedia object retrieval is becoming popular is of utmost importance to allow the user to formulate query which consist not only of a multimedia object, but at the same time –a textual or voice description.

Methods for measuring Quality of Experience

The introduction of more complex search methods than the users are used to create a new problem – the user perceived satisfaction and the method of its measurement.

When issuing a multimedia query it is hard to judge whether the result is relevant, and, furthermore whether the user will be satisfied with such result. The situation encountered here is much more complex than with traditional textual queries, as the opinion regarding the relevance of the query result will vary from user to user depending on the query context.

The information on the level of satisfaction of the user with a search service is critical, both during the development and deployment stages. A common methodology and toolbox for measurement of the Quality of Experience of search services would be also an aid for the academic community allowing for comparison of results achieved by different search engines.

4.1 Future Research Challenges

Defining the next generation of media search technologies requires major research efforts in multimedia, multimodal and deformable objects search. Indeed, the continuous and rapid growth of multimedia content available on the Internet has not been accompanied by a similar development of efficient, multimodal and intuitive cross media search capabilities.

Despite the significant achievements, the current technology suffers from a number of strong limitations which prevent the user to efficiently access the desired (and theoretically available) information. This leads to several research challenges which are grouped below in three interlaced categories:

Towards truly multimodal search

A first Research Challenge in this domain consists of the expansion of current schemes to truly multimodal capabilities (e.g. exploiting all information of all available modalities when searching for media content). When current search engines are mostly limited to text queries, future search engines will need to use richer and more diverse sources of information including combined data from speech, audio, video, images, 3D, social tags (either automatically or user generated), physiological signals providing information of the emotional state or activity of the user (heart beat, brain waves, etc) or geolocation information. An important aspect of this research challenge is the possibility of performing cross-modality search such as for example audio-based video retrieval (a typical example of the latter would be to retrieve a video –e.g. sequence of images - that semantically matches a given audio content such as music).

Other key aspects in multimodal search include the management of diversity and uncertainty in search to achieve richer and more personalized results, and the use of contextual information as a way to create a common ground to model the relationships among different content sources.

This challenge calls for new paradigms for content-based high-level (or semantic) signal representations that would permit cross modal navigation. It also appears obvious that major challenges remain in the field of machine learning and in particular with respect to multiple heterogeneous signals fusion, content and context adaptation using limited training data, and audio source separation. Finally, it is necessary to increase the quality of search by eliminating or grouping all multimedia content that does not add extra information to the user (because it is duplicated or of less quality than existing content) and implementing personalized search systems.

Towards search of multimodal and deformable content

Another important research challenge will target the access of complex, possibly multimodal and deformable information from a rudimentary query.

Indeed, current search experiences may be very tedious and especially in the case where it is not straightforward to describe the searched information with simple text queries. It is, here, highly desirable to be able to define a query by associating rudimentary and imperfect – possibly cross modal- descriptions of the searched information (e.g. search from hand drawn sketches, query by humming or low quality audio recordings, search for multiple videos of the same scene - but taken from different angles - search of 3D objects from 2D views or simple drawings or search of 2D projections of an object from the relevant 3D description, possibly considering 3D deformation models). This represents major theoretic research challenges in multi-level hierarchical content representation, in complex multimodal scene analysis and in decomposition models on known or unknown dictionaries or object bases.

Towards efficient user interaction

The third research challenge directly targets the development of new paradigms for *user interaction* (and satisfaction) in a multimodal context. It is, indeed, essential that future generation search tools can propose intuitive and rich query interfaces (multimodal, multi-level – that range from a full picture or only sketch – and intuitive

– e.g. by means of, for example, natural language), efficient presentation of the retrieved results and finally efficient means for user interaction with the retrieved information for successive searches. This includes the possibility of multimodal navigation across different media, for instance, jumping from a piece of soundtrack to the relevant movie, and then to other movies involving the same actor or to the e-book version of the book from which the movie originated.

It is critical to develop methods and tools for assessment of the quality of experience of the user. These methods were developed and standardized for voice and video services – now need to be moved forward to 3D content and multimedia services. This will put the user in the center of attention and will forge a true user-centric media environment.

This represents major challenges for the characterization of mono-modal and cross modal media similarity and its use in the selection of the retrieved information. Other research challenges of the same kind include the presentation of the retrieved information on heterogeneous devices and better user-feedback exploitation for multi query search in a fully multimodal context.

5   Content with Memory and Behaviour

In the area of 3D, virtual worlds and gaming, advances are needed to increase the level of realism and interactivity. By adding to virtual characters and virtual objects memory and behavior will lead to the transition from the "smart content" to the "intelligent content". The positioning and the advantages of the intelligent content may be seen in the following figure

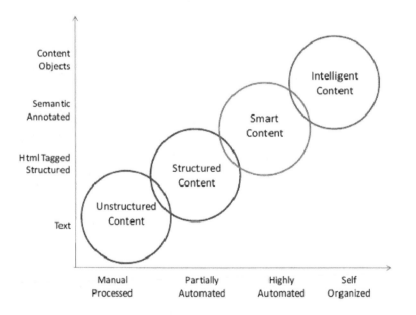

Fig. 4. Intelligent Content Positioning

We define as *Content Objects* polymorphic/holistic containers, which may consist of media, rules, behaviour, relations and characteristics or any combination of the above. *Media* can be anything that a human can perceive/experience with his/her senses, *characteristics* are meaningfully descriptions of the object, *Rules* refer to the way an object is treated and manipulated by other objects or the environment (discovered, retrieved, casted, adapted, delivered, transformed, presented), *behaviour* can refer to the way the object affects other objects or the environment, *relations* between an object with other objects can refer to time, space and synchronisation issues. As can be seen the integration of memory and behavior to content objects can in some sense be said to be the equivalent of personality for virtual characters. The behavior rules their interactions, while memory provides them with the capacity to remember past interactions and to learn from their experiences. As a result these virtual characters can interact socially and serve as companions for people and even potentially amongst each other. While the level of physical realism of these characters has vastly improved (improved movement, more realistic facial gestures, etc.), the biggest challenge not only making them look like humans but make them behave as natural as humans for which they must have social and cognitive intelligence, emotions and memory. To date this level of realism has not been achieved in any virtual worlds or games. The only characters which, today, have such a high level of social and cognitive skills are those which have a human being behind them. But providing emotions and personality for virtual characters isn't just a challenge for virtual worlds and gaming – it can have real world benefits in areas such as education and health care.

5.1 Future Research Challenges

Future Media must build on the new capabilities offered by new web technologies to provide an improved user experience. Content will adapt to user context and purpose. Such content exposes 'a behaviour'. It remembers, reacts, interacts and thereby actually becomes bi-directionally immersive, i.e. immerses the user as well as immerses itself into the user's environment.

Recent years brought us neologisms such as blobjects, blogjects, tweetjects and the Spime. All these terms denote a kind of object which is capable to converse with its environment – the real one as well as the virtual one. This is not just the Internet of things. Today, the Simple Object Access Protocol (SOAP) talks to systems, but in the future we will access objects – no matter what systems manage those objects or where they are managed.

Future Media will be composed of such autonomous content objects or content object mash-ups. The autonomous objects will *travel over the network, split and combine* to generate the new service or a 'virtual world object'.

The above ideas include a number of research challenges that have already been described. For example media encoding, media search etc. Yet, there is a number of research areas related to the content objects themselves:

Ontologies and Semantic Description

This set of challenge includes research on the modeling and semantic description of the content objects as media containers, along with descriptions of their structure, characteristics, behavior, rules and relations.

Decomposition and Reconstruction

This set of challenges includes research on the decomposition of scenes and scenarios, along with real-time component-preserving capturing technologies: advanced capturing systems using stereoscopic cameras, camera arrays, time-of-flight cameras or 3D scanners preserve three-dimensional information and thereby the components and their spatio-temporal relationships. Moreover, assembly and reconstruction of complex scenes and scenarios as content objects mash-ups.

Network Support for Content Objects

This set of challenges includes research on the network architecture (including distributed network intelligence, network topology and traffic awareness, content distribution including caches), and issues like routing and streaming of the content objects.

6 New Application Areas

The influence of the Internet in today's interpersonal communication and interaction with information has reached a level never imagined by past generations. The penetration of Internet services and applications has reached a stage that is starting to have a profound impact on different dimensions of people's lifestyles, including their everyday habits. The advances in Future Media technologies will enable innovative applications and services, engaging new experiences, where multimedia digital content will be more immersive and closely related to the physical world. In fact, the Future Internet will allow a new generation of online ubiquitous applications sustained by new enablers of the Internet amongst which the Internet of Services, the Internet of Things, the Internet of Media & Content and the Social Internet (see figure below).

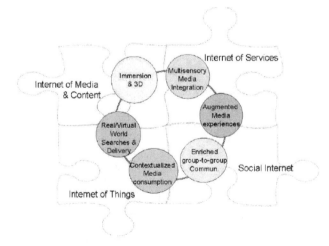

Fig. 5. New Dimensions of Applications Enablers of Future Internet

On top of these new dimensions of the Internet, the applications that will be created will allow users to enhance human-media and human-human communications as follows:

Immersive and 3D Applications

The envisioned new applications in this field will include revolutionary ways of interacting with media through sophisticated representations of real and virtual worlds. Among the kind of applications enabled by immersive media it is expected the appearance of new physically strong experiences such as exertion games, simulation and training of real life situations in realistic way (e.g. chirurgical interventions), new entertainment experiences (e.g. tele-reality concerts), and personal enriched communications (e.g. sophisticated tele-presence).

Multisensory Media Integration

The Future Internet will enable applications dealing not only with data and information but also will enhance the perception of digital contents by exploring new ways of impacting Human perception. In fact the Future Internet will include a new set of revolutionary applications focusing on enriching Human sensations. This will be achieved by stimulating simultaneously the different senses beyond audiovisual content by including haptics or smell.

Augmented Media Experiences

A set of new applications of the Future Internet is envisioned to impact the way people interact with the physical world. In fact, there are expected applications dealing with augmented media that will enrich elements in the physical world with digital content in a way that will modify the conception of reality. In such context, a new kind of reality will be conceived as the sum of physical and augmented information that will go beyond early augmented reality prototypic developments into a well established discipline rich of applications and services.

Enriched Group to Group Communications

Traditional one-to-one and group-to-group communications will be transformed in the context of the Future Internet. The kind of applications envisioned in this concern, will include synchronous and asynchronous interactions including multi-channel sources to enhance the way people communicate.

Typical applications and services in this domain will include engaging of distant family members into end-to-end games and collaborative work with remotely located teams, involving verbal and nonverbal communications and interaction with tangible devices and objects.

Contextualized Media Consumptions

Future Media will enable applications where information not only will be available at any time but moreover its consumption will be adaptive in order to be selective in terms of when, where and how to present it.

This will imply a level of intelligence embedded in media and in its composition in order that users will be able to access content in its best possible way and in the right moment when it is needed. This will allow for applications contextualized according to personal profiles, location, types of media, available devices, resources and QoS needs.

Real-Virtual Worlds Searches and Delivery

The Future Internet will include a rich set of applications dealing with real, virtual and mixed information and consequently its identification and retrieval. The envisioned applications in this respect will include searching facilities allowing for cross modal search in both, input and output. This means that the input mechanisms enabled by search applications will allow not only textual queries but also multimodal ones while the output will be given also in combined modalities. Moreover, the searches will not be limited to the virtual world but will retrieve information regarding physical objects, their location, their state and their relationship and enrichment with digital contents.

7 Conclusion

This paper has presented a series of new research trends for the design and study of Future User-Centric Media technology. As a result of previous discuss sessions among experts coordinated by the FMI-TF, research challenges were identified and highlighted with the goal of determining the current trend and future perspectives of the research community on the Future Media technology, with emphasis on their impact and potential application in the area of Ambient Systems and Media.

References

1. Nokia Research Center, Extended Home Team,
   http://research.nokia.com/extendedhome/
2. Orb, http://www.orb.com/
3. IST Amigo Project, Deliverable D2.2: State of the art analysis including assessment of system architectures for ambient intelligence (April 2005)
4. IST ePerSpace Project, Report of State of the Art in Personalisation. Common Framework (February 2004)
5. IST ePerSpace Project, D4.1: Content Management Architecture design (November 2004)
6. CONTENT D2.1 Deliverable CONTENT Research Vision and Roadmap (March 2007), http://www.istcontent.eu

Author Index